Numeracy, Clinical Calculations and Basic Statistics

A Textbook for Health Care Students

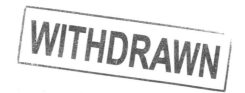

Numeracy, Clinical Calculations and Basic Statistics

A Textbook for Health Care Students

Neil Davison

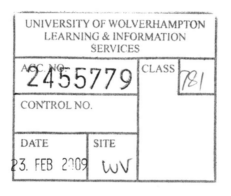
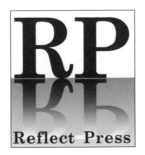

Reflect Press

First published in 2008

ISBN: 978 1 906052 07 2

British Library Cataloguing in Publication Data
A catalogue record for this book is available from the British Library

The author and publisher have made every attempt to ensure the content of this book is up to date and accurate. However, health care knowledge and information is changing all the time so the reader is advised to double-check any information in this text on drug usage, calculations, treatment procedures, the use of equipment, etc. to confirm that it complies with the latest safety recommendations, standards of practice and legislation, as well as local Trust policies and procedures. Students are advised to check with their tutor and/or mentor before carrying out the procedures in this textbook and all drug calculations must be checked by a Registered Practitioner before drugs are administered to a patient.

Production project management by Deer Park Productions

Typeset by PDQ Typesetting

Cover design by Oxmed

Printed and bound by Cromwell Press Ltd, Trowbridge, Wiltshire

Distributed by BEBC, Albion Close, Parkstone, Poole, Dorset BH12 3LL

Published by Reflect Press Ltd
11 Attwyll Avenue
Exeter
Devon, EX2 5HN
UK
01392 204400
www.reflectpress.com

Contents

Introduction

This book is designed and written for student nurses, registered nurses and other health care professionals. Nurses undertaking 'return to practice' and 'adaptation' courses will find the contents of the book useful as the expectations of these courses are similar to those of pre-registration nursing programmes. Students currently on further education 'BTEC National Diploma' and 'Access to Higher Education' courses, who are planning a career in health care, will also find the content relevant.

If you are a student nurse, you will be aware of the need to perform calculations accurately and that the failure to compute the correct answer 100 per cent of the time could harm members of the public. This responsibility can cause anxieties and self-doubt. However, by reading this book you have started to address these issues. The book will provide opportunities to practise and develop the numeracy skills needed for safe clinical practice.

If you are a registered nurse you may have concerns about interpreting research findings or, if you are planning to change jobs, you could encounter a numeracy test as part of the selection process. You may also be unsure about the expectations of future students in your clinical area who need to develop and demonstrate their numeracy skills as part of the Nursing and Midwifery Council's (NMC's) Essential Skill Clusters. If you are facing any of these issues, or you simply want to maintain your current numeracy and calculation skills, then read on.

When it comes to mathematics, people can be grouped into 'those who can' and 'those who think they can't' (Lerwill, 1999). A great deal of our anxiety about mathematics comes down to a lack of confidence. This book will help to develop your confidence by giving you the fundamentals of arithmetic needed for calculating in the health care environment, by developing a thorough understanding of the units of measurement currently used, and by providing formulae for calculating drug dosages. Later chapters explore the use of numeric scales in health care and introduce some basic statistical concepts and measurements that are prerequisites when reading research.

The book is designed so that you don't have to progress through the chapters in the order that they are written. Some readers will want to start at Chapter One and study through to Chapter Six, but some will want to dip into the chapter that has most relevance for them at that time. In each chapter, topics are introduced and the relevance to clinical practice is made clear. There are regular opportunities to test your understanding of the topic before you progress to the next one. Collectively the chapters will provide a numeracy knowledge base for clinical practice, improve your confidence with calculations and help you to prepare to get the most from clinical placements and experience.

Author biography

Neil Davison is a Lecturer in Nursing and Teaching Fellow at Bangor University. During his clinical career, Neil trained and worked in Shropshire, Herefordshire and Lincolnshire, specialising in orthopaedic and trauma nursing. His interest in numeracy and nursing calculations has developed from teaching student nurses to calculate drug dosages and from his role as an Admissions Tutor trying to ensure that applicants have the required numeracy skills to become safe registered nurses.

Dedication

This book was inspired by the lives of Arnold J. Davison and Donald E.W. Makepeace, two great men who taught me that there is always a solution.

Chapter 1

The need for numeracy and calculation skills in the clinical environment

INTRODUCTION

This chapter provides an overview of the current issues relating to nurses' numeracy skills. It explores the failings of numeracy skills in nurses, and discusses the impact that these failings could have in clinical practice. Current professional standards for numeracy are explored and the methods that students can use to develop and improve their numeracy skills are outlined. Finally the chapter considers the future and how this may impact on nurses' numeracy skills.

THE PROBLEMS WITH NURSES AND NUMBERS

There are concerns about the ability of nurses to accurately calculate drug dosages (Jukes and Gilchrist, 2006). This could be perceived as a recent problem, possibly resulting from the methods used to teach **mathematics** within the general education system. The reality is somewhat different. Failings in nurses' **numeracy** skills and the effect that these may have on the safe administration of medicines have been raised consistently over the last two decades, and featured in the literature as far back as 1939 (Weeks, Lyne and Torrance, 2000). Also, concerns about nurses' numeracy skills are not confined to the UK. Cartwright (1996) outlined similar problems in America, Canada, Australia and New Zealand.

Whittaker (1987) wrote about innumerate nurses who needed additional education and support to help in the accurate calculation of drug dosages. Miller (1992) added to the debate, reiterating doubts about the mathematical skills of nurses. Hutton (2000, p. 894) described nurses as being 'typical of the population as a whole in that many are not good at numerical calculations'. By 2004 the state of nurses' drug calculation skills was the focus of national concern (Department of Health, 2004a). Mistakes in the prescribing and administration of drugs account for 25% of litigation claims in the UK (Department of Health, 2004a). Worryingly, the government pledge to reduce this by 40% (Department of Health, 2000) has not been achieved. The available research and literature, as well as governmental and professional reports and policy, indicate that over the last two decades there has been an acceptance that, for whatever reason, there is a problem with nurses' numeracy skills, and there is unlikely to be one simple solution.

THE NEED FOR NUMERACY AND CALCULATION SKILLS IN THE HEALTH CARE ENVIRONMENT

It may seem obvious that nurses need to have good numeracy skills, but this has been debated in the literature. Cartwright (1996) was unconvinced that the safe administration of drugs demanded that nurses have mathematical skills, but did accept that these skills would be needed for other aspects of nurses' roles such as, for example, applying the results of research to practice. Hutton (1998), Sandwell and Carson (2005) and Jukes and Gilchrist (2006) all accept that mathematical skills are essential in nursing.

The NMC view numeracy skills as a fundamental aspect of the role of the nurse, and this extends beyond the administration of drugs to include nutritional and fluid measurements. The recently announced **Essential Skills Clusters** (NMC, 2007a) demand that students who start an educational programme leading to registration from September 2008 will have their numeracy skills assessed. This means that, to become a registered nurse, students will be assessed during the first year of their educational programme to enable progression to Branch. During a practice placement in the Branch programme, students must achieve 100% in a test of their numeracy skills to be able to register with the NMC.

The consequences of inadequate numeracy skills

Shortcomings in nurses' numeracy skills are related to medication errors, with wrong doses commonly associated with nurses' miscalculations (Department of Health, 2004b). There is evidence that nurses do have problems with calculations and, in particular, with performing some basic procedures like long division and multiplication (Wright, 2006). Beyond drug administration, there are many other calculations performed in clinical practice but these rarely feature in the literature or seem to give cause for concern. Poor calculation ability can lead to drug errors (Wright, 2006), but the exact number of mistakes attributable to miscalculations isn't known. What is known is that drug dose calculations are one of a series of steps in the administration of medicines and, as health care professionals, nurses and midwives should ensure that each of these is

performed to the highest possible standard, and that any risk to the recei-
ver of the medication is reduced to an absolute minimum.

The reality of clinical practice is a complex mixture of skills underpinned
by relevant theory. Accurate drug calculations are dependent on more
than numeracy skills, because they also involve an understanding of how
drug doses are presented, and the units of measurement used within
clinical practice. Competency in performing basic calculations is a fundamental aspect of drug administration. Errors with decimal points can lead
to mistakes in administration (Department of Health, 2000), and are also
a frequent cause of prescribing mistakes (Department of Health, 2004a),
which nurses need to be on the lookout for, and need to resolve, before
the drug can be administered. The ways that drug dosages are expressed
varies from dilution (1 in 1000), mass concentration (1 mg in 1 ml) to
percentage concentrations (0.1%), which make for complex calculations,
a known source of error (Department of Health, 2004a).

Failing to carefully record everyday clinical measurements can also lead to
errors. A mistake in the recording of a patient's body weight in pounds
instead of kilograms led to a drug calculation error where the dosage was
calculated per kilogram of body weight (Department of Health, 2000).
The complexity of clinical practice and the importance of each aspect of
care are tragically illustrated by a Fatal Accident and Sudden Death
Inquiry held in Scotland in November 2005. A nurse administered 40
units of insulin instead of the prescribed 4 units. She failed to get her
dosage calculation checked by a colleague. The poor-quality handwriting
of another nurse led to the miscalculation, and a failure to measure and
record the patient's blood sugar and monitor her condition after the
administration all contributed to the patient's death.

Having painted a fairly complex and bleak picture, don't get down-
hearted about this, or spend too much time and energy ensuring that
you can perform all manner of calculations. It is obviously important to
be accurate, but the reality is that drug administration errors are more
often caused by a failure to perform the basic checks, including the drug,
route, time and patient (Cooper, 1995), than because of a calculation
error. You may take some comfort from Hutton (2000, p. 894), who
believes that 'Most nurses learn by experience to become competent in
the mathematical calculations they perform and to know what is a
reasonable dose.' Reading this book is part of your learning experience
as you are learning from the experiences and, unfortunately, the mistakes
of other nurses.

PROFESSIONAL STANDARDS FOR NUMERACY

For several years the NMC has set standards for numeracy that applicants need to achieve prior to starting a pre-registration nursing course. These vary from national qualifications like GCSE mathematics at grade C or above, or Key Skills Level Two 'Application of Number', to locally developed tests designed by individual universities. During pre-registration nursing and midwifery courses, students are required to use their numeracy skills to demonstrate that they can safely administer medicines and that they can interpret numerical data and use this in the safe delivery of care (NMC, 2004). Recently, the NMC has reviewed pre-registration nursing programmes and has announced the Essential Skills Clusters (NMC, 2007a). These are skills statements aimed at complementing the outcomes and proficiencies that students have to achieve, and are targeted on aspects of care that, if not performed competently, would put patients at risk. From a numeracy perspective, the skills clusters make it clear that the ability to perform calculations and interpret data go considerably further than administering medicines and include baseline patient assessments and nutritional and fluid support. The NMC plays a major role in protecting members of the public. Setting standards for registration and demanding that your numeracy skills will be assessed where you will use them, in clinical practice, should mean that both you and the public have confidence in your ability.

Using electronic calculators in practice

The use of an electronic calculator is an accepted part of modern life and, for many people, it is an essential tool to ensure accuracy. The NMC caution nurses about the place of calculators when making drug calculations:

> The use of calculators to determine the volume or quantity of medication should not act as a substitute for **arithmetical** knowledge and skill.
>
> (NMC, 2007b, p. 24)

This may seem an odd view to take and cause you some concern. Don't get too worried about this, as many students initially feel anxious that they won't be able to cope without a calculator. It could be assumed that using a calculator increases accuracy in calculations and, therefore, reduces the risk of error. However, this doesn't take into account the fact that, in order to safely calculate complex drug doses, it is essential to have an understanding of the basic mathematical principles involved, as well as an ability to estimate an answer. Estimation involves 'mental maths' and provides the parameters within which the exact answer will lie. For example, if a calculation involved 5 multiplied by 4.5, an estimate would tell you that the answer lies between 5 x 4 and 5 x 5, which equal 20 and 25. Estimation is a critical stage in calculating drug doses as it can prevent large mistakes that may occur through decimal point errors. The guidance offered by the NMC doesn't prevent the checking of a drug calculation by a second nurse with a calculator, nor does it state that calculations other than medication calculations cannot be performed using a calculator.

One of the major problems facing many health care students is that they are products of an education system that may have actively encouraged a dependence upon a calculator. Because of changes to the teaching of numeracy and mathematics in both primary and secondary education, there will be nurses who can perform drug calculations with or without a calculator, and there will be those who cannot operate without the assistance of a calculator (Pentin and Smith, 2006). If you consider yourself to be a member of the latter group don't despair, because this book will become part of your strategy to improve both your competence and confidence with calculations.

OPPORTUNITIES TO DEVELOP YOUR NUMERACY AND CALCULATION SKILLS

One of the fundamental ways of improving any skill is by practice and repetition. However, there are suggestions that the frequency and number of calculations that nurses need to perform have decreased, effectively deskilling nurses (Hutton, 1998). This may be partially attributed to the technological developments of electronic drip rate counters and volumetric infusion pumps that calculate infusion flow rates. An additional obstacle for some nursing students is the development of single nurse drug administration. In some circumstances, such as the administration of intravenous preparations or controlled drugs, where complex calculations are needed, or where the administration is to a child, two nurses are still required. In practice this does mean that there are many occasions where a registered nurse doesn't need a student to check and witness the administration of medicines, resulting in a reduction in the opportunities for practising numeracy skills. It is important for you to be aware of this, so that you can take advantage of any situation involving drug administration and calculations.

In aiming to achieve confidence and competence in numeracy skills, there are obstacles to overcome, but there is a great deal that individual students can do to ensure their personal success and the safety of patients. Numeracy skills are an essential clinical skill, so think about where and how you may achieve their development. If you are allocated to a surgical ward for a placement, you will have probably spent some time before starting work considering which **clinical outcomes** can be best practised and achieved within a surgical environment. Treat numeracy and calculation skills the same way. If you are unsure of the learning opportunities available or how these might allow you to practise calculations, talk to the **Link Tutor** from your university and/or other students who may have spent time on a surgical placement. Ideally, visit the ward and meet with your **mentor** before starting on the placement. The ward may produce a booklet for students outlining typical learning opportunities. Aim to make the most of every minute of your clinical experience. Working alongside an experienced nurse and getting involved in drug rounds will help you to develop the required calculation skills, as well as helping you to become familiar with common drug doses and to recognise when something isn't right.

In preparation for clinical placements, many skills are learned and practised away from the clinical environment, usually in a classroom or skills laboratory setting. Numeracy and calculation skills can also be developed by this method but, first, it is necessary to consider what fundamental numeracy skills are used when calculating drug doses and other clinically related numeracy activities. An understanding of, and ability to use, the fundamental mathematical principles of addition, subtraction, multiplication, division, fractions and decimals have been identified as essential for calculating drug dosages (Wright, 2006). Within clinical areas, the use of numeracy skills extends beyond drug calculations, as they are required for many aspects of daily clinical activities like fluid balance measurements and dependency scores. Clinical calculations usually involve a unit of measurement such as litres, so students also need to be familiar with the common measurement units used. Also, educational programmes leading to registration and the modern health care environment dictate that nurses are able to read and interpret research studies, which places additional demands on numeracy skills.

Revision of your previous learning about mathematics (Wright, 2006), particularly if this is made relevant to nursing, is thought to be valuable in enhancing numeracy skills, as well as the use of self-instructional texts (Hutton, 1998). If you glance briefly at the contents page of this book, you will see that it offers coverage of all of the key stages needed to develop your numeracy skills. Chapter Two reviews the mathematical principles you will need and Chapter Three explores the units of measurement used in clinical practice. Later chapters consider other calculations used in practice and help you prepare to venture into some basic statistical issues.

NUMERACY SKILLS IN THE FUTURE

Numeracy skills are similar to all academic and clinical skills in that they need periodic updating. Don't be tempted to think that you can forget about them beyond initial registration. With the modernisation of health services and nursing career developments, it is likely that, in future, many more nurses will be prescribing drugs. A significant part of being a prescriber is demonstrating accuracy in calculations. There have also been attempts to assess the numeracy skills of health care professionals, including nurses, prior to employment. The *Daily Telegraph* (Hall, 5 August 2006) reported that the East Kent NHS Trust in Canterbury was using a numeracy test as part of a selection process. Whether activities like this are based on a genuine concern for nurses' numeracy skills and patient safety, or are part of a way of rationing nurses' posts in a time of shortage, remains to be seen. There could be a possibility that, in future, NHS Trusts may want to test the numeracy skills of all health professionals employed within a Trust. Before starting along this path, the full implications of discovering that some health professionals can't pass a numeracy test needs detailed consideration. This could lead to considerable public alarm and a lack of confidence in local health services, as well as requiring significant financial resources to correct.

Activity

Numeracy skills review
Hopefully reading this chapter has raised some issues that will make you take a critical but balanced look at your own numeracy skills. The aim of the checklist below is to draw attention to the skills and knowledge that are commonly put into practice in the health care environment. This should act as a reminder of those of your skills that need further development and practice. The remainder of this book and your clinical experience will ensure that you are in the best position to meet the required professional standards for your future career.

- Can you perform the following basic principles of mathematics accurately?
    - Addition.
    - Subtraction.
    - Multiplication.
    - Division.
- Are you familiar with metric units of measurement?
- Are you confident in the use of decimal points?
- Are you confident in the use of fractions?
- Do you have recent, regular experience of using numbers and performing calculations?

Activity

Preparation for clinical placement

After you receive the details of your practice placement allocation, start planning the ways in which your clinical experience will develop your numeracy and calculation skills. Give some thought to potential situations where your numeracy skills will be used. Possibilities include:

- Admitting patients and performing baseline assessments and observations. Patients might expect you to be able to convert their body weight from kilograms into stones and pounds.
- Administering medicines means you will have the opportunity to work with experienced nurses and observe how they perform calculations.
- Patients who are having their fluid intake and output recorded will provide you with the experience of measuring and recording fluids, as well as performing calculations.

SUMMARY
- Nurses need to be competent calculators to enable the safe administration of medicines.
- Numeracy skills are essential for many other areas of practice like completing fluid balance charts and enabling evidence-based practice through the interpretation of research results.
- Electronic calculators can be useful in checking a calculation, but should not be substituted for an understanding of the basic rules of mathematics.
- Remember that while accuracy is crucial when performing calculations, there are other sources of error when administering medicines.
- Keep a balanced approach to developing your numeracy skills and don't invest all of your time calculating drug dosages to the neglect of other areas of study.

FURTHER READING

Pentin, J. and Smith, J. (2006) 'Drug calculations: are they safer with or without a calculator?' *British Journal of Nursing,* 15(14): 778–81
This article explores the issues surrounding the use of calculators in the safe administration of medicines. Problems with nurses' numeracy skills are discussed, and the role that the general education system has played is outlined. The implications for patient safety are explored and ways that

nurses can develop and maintain proficiency with calculations are discussed.

Medicines Management. Available from the 'A-Z of Advice' link at The Nursing and Midwifery Council website, **www.nmc-uk.org**
This guidance provides essential information about all aspects of drug administration for nurses and midwives. The principles of administering drugs are discussed and advice about performing calculations and the role of electronic calculators is provided. This resource contains a lot of information that students and registered nurses will find valuable.

Essential Skills Clusters. An overview of the content and purpose of the Essential Skills Clusters can be found on the NMC website at:
www.nmc-uk.org/aFrameDisplay.aspx?DocumentID=2618
Further details are contained in an additional document available at:
www.nmc-uk.org/aFrameDisplay.aspx?DocumentID=2690
Together, these documents give an indication of the aspects of nursing that require numeracy skills and are likely to be assessed in clinical practice.

Chapter 2

Back to Basics

INTRODUCTION

This chapter begins with a basic introduction to the decimal system. The need to be able to work in numbers greater as well as less than one is discussed. The role of digits and zeros within a number is explored and the purpose of the decimal point is identified. The four basic methods of calculating – addition, subtraction, multiplication and division – are then reviewed, and the use and calculation of percentages is explained. Fractions are considered as a way of breaking down numbers and expressing quantities less than one. The use of powers in the health care environment is discussed as a method of expressing large numbers.

NUMBERS AND DIGITS

An understanding of **decimals** and ability to work with them is essential in the clinical environment. Most people are comfortable with whole numbers such as 11, 250 and 975, but it is also necessary to be able to work in smaller units, or **fractions** of one. Some medications are prescribed using apparently large numbers like, for example, Paracetamol 500 mg, and some are prescribed in amounts that include fractions of one like, for example, the diuretic agent Bendrofluazide 2.5 mg. It is often units smaller than one that create anxiety, but it is worth considering what larger numbers mean as this helps in the understanding of numbers written to the right of the decimal point.

The decimal system

A number is made up from individual digits and communicates a great deal of information. If 625 is used as an example, this isn't simply a '6', a '2' and a '5'. The place of the number within the sequence gives a value and, reading from left to right, 625 has a value of 6 'hundreds', 2 'tens' and 5 'ones'. This is because we use a 'base 10' decimal system. The basis of this system is that each number is ten times greater than the number to the right of it. Equally, numbers are ten times smaller than the number to their left. Figure 2.1 presents this visually.

MILLIONS	HUNDRED THOUSANDS	TEN THOUSANDS	THOUSANDS	HUNDREDS	TENS	ONES / UNITS	DECIMAL POINT	TENTHS	HUNDREDTHS	THOUSANDTHS
1 000 000	100 000	10 000	1 000	100	10	1	.	0.1	0.01	0.001
6	5	4	3	2	1		.	1	2	3

Whole numbers to the left   Decimal point   Decimal fractions to the right

Figure 1 Whole numbers and decimal fractions

The role of zero

Within the decimal system, zeros play an important role when there are no unit values. If the number 605 is used as an example, '6' indicates six hundreds, '0' indicates no tens and '5' indicates five ones. The '0' maintains the position of the other digits within the number. One-digit numbers range from 1 to 9, two-digit numbers range from 10 to 99, three-digit numbers range from 100 to 999, four-digit numbers range from 1 000 to 9 999 and so on.

When writing numbers that contain four digits or more, there is a convention to use a comma or gap within the number to make it easier to read. One thousand can be written as 1,000 or 1 000. This book uses the gap convention, as this is standard within the metric (SI) system used in health care.

Removing trailing zeros

Zeros can maintain the position of other digits, but they can also be the source of error. When administering medications or fluids, it is critical to remove any trailing zeros. These are zeros that are used after the decimal point and don't maintain the position of other digits within a number. This can be illustrated with the drug dose of 5 mg. This should be written as 5 mg and not 5.0 mg because if the decimal point is not seen the result is a huge overdose. Trailing zeros have been identified as a potential source of serious drug errors (Department of Health, 2004a).

The decimal point

If whole numbers are written, the decimal point is omitted, but when a number includes a fraction of one (a decimal fraction), the decimal point is used to signpost the extent of the whole number and the start of the decimal fraction. This practice is common in the health care environment. For example, a nurse could be part time and work 30 hours per week or full time and work 37.5 hours per week. Although the role of decimal points may seem theoretical, it is vital that you understand this as the position of the decimal point is recognised as a potential source of serious drug administration errors (Department of Health, 2004a).

Self-assessment progress check

Digit value
The recap questions below will help to consolidate your learning about the value of digits within a number. The answers can be found on page 83.

1. In the number 20 641, what value does the '6' have?
2. In the number 102 003, what value does the '2' have?
3. In the number 342 970, what value does the '3' have?
4. In the number 17.45, what value does the '5' have?
5. In the number 1.025, what value does the '0' have?
6. In the number 6.005, what value does the '5' have?
7. In the number 70.648, what value does the '6' have?
8. In the number 10.289, what value does the '0' have?
9. In the number 135.008, what value does the '3' have?
10. In the number 0.02, what value does the '2' have?

Practice tip
Don't assume that it is only drug dosages that demand accuracy. All numbers need to be read carefully, by double-checking the positions of zeros and the decimal point, as these are known sources of error. A decimal point mistake will make a large difference to any number, whether this is the output from a wound drain or a baby's body weight. Remember that clinical decisions may be based partly on your assessments and observations, so they have to be accurate.

METHODS OF CALCULATING

Numbers are a part of everyday life, including working out the super-market bill, calculating how many miles per gallon your car is achieving and making sure that your payslip is correct. Depending on the size of the numbers, calculations can be done mentally, on paper or with a calculator. Irrespective of how the calculations are made, the basic methods are the same and nurses (and other health care professionals) need to be able to perform these. The NMC (2007b) have cautioned that calculators are no substitute for arithmetical knowledge and skill. It is worth remembering that to use a calculator accurately, a sound understanding of the decimal system and the four basic calculation methods – addition, subtraction, multiplication and division – is required.

Addition

Most simple additions can be calculated mentally but, where many individual numbers have to be added together like, for example, when calculating the fluid intake of a patient over 24 hours, the potential for errors increases. In these circumstances it is sensible to perform the calculation on paper. This is when an understanding of the basics of the decimal system is useful and when it is necessary to remember that individual digits within a number have a value – ones, tens, hundreds or greater.

The numbers are written down in a column format as in the example below. The columns are not usually labelled as hundreds (h), tens (t) or ones, but this helps to illustrate the calculation. Of course, if this method suits you, then use it. When adding two or more numbers together, the calculation can be performed in any order: 74 + 26 gives the same answer as 26 + 74.

As well as an ability to add two or more numbers together, you also need to be able to check that you haven't made a basic error with your calculation. Remember that if you add numbers together, your answer must be greater than the numbers that you started with.

Example 1

```
h  t  ones
6  2  5 +
   7  2
6  9  7
```

Method
The addition is calculated vertically from right to left, starting under the 'ones' column, and involves three individual calculations, one for the 'ones' column, one for the 'tens' column' and a final calculation for the 'hundreds' column.

Process
Starting with the 'ones' column:
5 + 2 = 7
Moving left to the 'tens' column:
2 + 7 = 9
Moving left to the 'hundreds' column:
6 + 0 = 6
This gives the answer of 6 hundreds, 9 tens and 7 ones, or 697.

Not all additions are this straightforward as there will be times when the calculation results in ten or more in a column, as in Example 2.

Example 2
h t ones
5 0 4 +
   ¹5 7
—————
5 6 1

Method
As before, the addition is calculated vertically from right to left, starting under the 'ones' column.

Process
Starting with the 'ones' column:
4 + 7 = 11

The number '11' is made up of one 'ten' and a single 'one'. As this column is only used to record the 'ones', the single 'one' is recorded here and the 'ten' carried over to the 'tens' column. The usual way of doing this is to write a small '1' by the 5 under the 'tens' column.

Moving left to the 'tens' column:
0 + 5 + 1 (carried over from the 'ones' column) = 6

Moving left to the 'hundreds' column:
5 + 0 = 5
This gives the answer of 5 hundreds, 6 tens and 1 ones, or 561.

If the addition involves more than two numbers, as it is likely to be when calculating a fluid balance record, the method and process are the same.

Self-assessment progress check

Addition

The recap questions below will help to consolidate your learning about additions. The answers can be found on page 83.

1.   795 +
     1 052

2.   9 726 +
     18 387

3.   501 +
     1 609

4.   206 016 +
     14 492

5.   175
     130
     50
     15
     430 +
     500

6.   15
     30
     45
     130
     150 +
     220

Subtraction

Subtraction involves the taking of one number from another and is frequently used in the calculation of fluid balance records to determine if the patient is in a negative or positive state of fluid balance. Subtraction is also used to calculate the stock levels of controlled drugs following administration.

It is vital that you understand which number is to be subtracted from the other, because if you get the numbers in the wrong order the calculation may appear confusing and will result in a strange answer. For example, 79 – 23 = 56, but 23 – 79 will give an answer that is less than zero, or a negative number.

The same basic rules apply as they did for addition: individual digits within a number have a value – ones, tens, hundreds or greater. As in any method of calculating, it is important that the digit positions are maintained to avoid errors and this is where the use of columns can help. Don't forget to check that you haven't made a basic error with your calculation. Remember that if you subtract, the answer must be less than the number that you started with.

have forgotten them, you might find that a copy of the 'multiplication grid' on page 28 acts as a valuable resource.

When multiplying two or more numbers together, the calculation can be performed in any order: 25 × 4 gives the same answer as 4 × 25.

Example 1

```
h  t  ones
1  2  3  ×
      3
_____
3  6  9
```

Method
The multiplication is calculated vertically from right to left, starting under the 'ones' column, and involves three individual calculations, one for the 'ones' column, one for the 'tens' column' and a final calculation for the 'hundreds' column.

Process
Starting with the 'ones' column:
3 × 3 = 9

Moving left to the 'tens' column:
3 × 2 = 6

Moving left to the 'hundreds' column:
3 × 1 = 3

This gives the answer of 3 hundreds, 6 tens and 9 ones, or 369.

Not all multiplications are as straightforward as this. There will be times when the calculation results in ten or more in a column, as in Example 2.

Example 2

```
h  t  ones
2  ¹2  4  ×
       4
_____
8  9  6
```

Method
As before, the multiplication is calculated vertically from right to left, starting under the 'ones' column, and involves three individual calculations, one for the 'ones' column, one for the 'tens' column' and a final calculation for the 'hundreds' column.

Process
Starting with the 'ones' column:
$4 \times 4 = 16$
The number '16' is made up of one 'ten' and six 'ones'. As this column is only used to record the 'ones', the six 'ones' are recorded here and the 'ten' carried over to the 'tens' column. The usual way of doing this is to write a small '1' by the 2 under the 'tens' column.

Moving left to the 'tens' column:
$4 \times 2 = 8$ plus the 1 which was carried over from the 'ones' column $= 9$

Moving left to the 'hundreds' column:
$4 \times 2 = 8$

This gives the answer of 8 hundreds, 9 tens and 6 ones, or 896.

This process works well when the multiplication involves one number that is less than ten. When both of the numbers to be multiplied together are greater than ten, an extra stage of calculation is necessary.

Example 3
A nurse on night duty works 11 hours each shift. Over the last eight weeks she has worked 23 shifts. Her contract states that she needs to work a minimum of 240 hours over this period. Has she worked enough hours? This calculation involves multiplying 23 and 11.

```
h   t   ones
    2   3 ×
    1   1
   _____
    2   3 +
2   3   0
_____
2   5   3
```

Method
As before, the multiplication is calculated vertically from right to left, making sure that individual digits are kept in position within the columns. The terms 'ones', 'tens' or 'hundreds' column used within the explanation only refer to the top number in the calculation.
Process
The multiplication has two stages, firstly multiplying the top number by the 1 'one' belonging to the 11 and secondly multiplying the top number by the 1 'ten' belonging to the 11.

Stage one
Starting with the 'ones' column:
$1 \times 3 = 3$

Moving left to the 'tens' column:
$1 \times 2 = 2$

Stage two
Stage two starts by placing a 'zero' under the 'ones' column to maintain the place of the other digits. This is done because the number being used in the multiplication from the bottom line is a ten, not a 'one'.

Starting with the 'ones' column:
$1 \times 3 = 3$ (but the answer is recorded under the 'tens' column as this is really $10 \times 3 = 30$)

Moving left to the 'tens' column:
$1 \times 2 = 2$ (but the answer is recorded under the 'hundreds' column as this is really $10 \times 20 = 200$)

The results of the two separate multiplications are then added together:
$23 + 230 = 253$

It also tells us that the night nurse worked more than enough hours!

Self-assessment progress check

Multiplication

The recap questions below will help to consolidate your learning about multiplication. The answers can be found on pages 83–84.

1.	18 ×
	  3
		2.	192 ×
			   4

3.	27 ×
	  9
		4.	691 ×
			  17

5.	74 ×
	  16
		6.	78 ×
			  24

Multiplying decimals

It will be necessary to be able to multiply decimals together and, although this is viewed as one of those awkward calculations, there is a simple trick to help get this right. Imagine that you had to calculate the annual leave entitlement for a member of staff. Nurse Williams is entitled to 2.5 days annual leave for each month that she works, but she has only worked on the ward for 3.5 months. To calculate the amount of annual leave that she can take means multiplying 3.5 (months) by 2.5 (days):

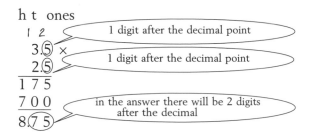

One of the problems encountered by many people is knowing where to put the decimal point. This is guided in two ways. Firstly it is necessary to perform an estimation of the likely answer. This isn't an exact calculation but should provide a rough guide to the real answer. You can estimate that 3 lots of 2.5 equal 7.5, and 4 lots of 2.5 are 10. We need an answer somewhere between these two values, so the only place that the decimal point can go is between the '8' and the '7' to make 8.75. Placing the decimal point in other positions would produce answers that are a long way from our estimation: 87.5 or 875. The second way of calculating where to place the decimal point is performed by adding up the number of digits to the right of the decimal point in the numbers being multiplied together. The upper number (3.5) has one digit after the decimal point and the lower number (2.5) has one digit after the decimal point. Adding these together gives 2, so there should be two digits after the decimal point in our final answer. Try this when multiplying decimals with several digits after the decimal point – it really does work.

Division

Dividing is a process that involves sharing. The first number is shared by a second number. This can also be thought of as 'how many times the second number will go into the first'. In the previous section, multiplication was said to be like repeated additions. In the same way division is like repeated subtractions. There are two symbols used to indicate that the calculation is a division: ÷ or one number placed above another, separated by a line –.

$32 \div 8 = 4$

or

$\dfrac{32}{8} = 4$

For example, there are 18 beds on the Medical admissions unit and six nurses on duty. To share out the workload equally, each nurse will have 3 beds to manage because:

$18 \div 6 = 3$

Divisions are frequently used to calculate the hourly flow rate of intravenous fluids administered to patients. Electronic infusion devices can calculate flow rates, but nurses need to be able to check any calculations in the event of a malfunction.

When calculating divisions, the method used is different to that used for additions, subtractions and multiplications in that the calculation starts with the left-hand number.

Example 1

$126 \div 3$

```
   h  t ones
      4 2
3/1  2 6
```

Method
The division is calculated from left to right, starting under the largest unit column, in this example 'hundreds'.

Process
Starting with the 'hundreds' column:
3 divided into 1 will not go because 1 is smaller than 3.
3 is now divided into 12, placing the result 4 above the line in the 'tens' column.

3 is now divided into the remaining 6 and the result placed above in the 'ones' column.

This gives the answer of 4 'tens' and 2 'ones', or 42.

Some divisions are more complex than this, as in Example 2.

Example 2

$138 \div 6$

```
  h  t  ones
        2  3
6/1  3  8
     ı
```

Method
The division is calculated from left to right, starting under the largest unit column – 'hundreds'.

Process
Starting with the 'hundreds' column:
6 divided into 1 will not go because 1 is smaller than 6.
6 is now divided into 13, placing the result 2 above the line in the 'tens' column, but this also leaves one 'ten' left over which is placed under the three in the 'tens' column.

6 is then divided into 18 (the one 'ten' remaining plus the eight 'ones') and the result 3 is placed above in the 'ones' column.

This gives the answer of 2 'tens' and 3 'ones', or 23.

Self-assessment progress check

Division

The recap questions below will help to consolidate your learning about division. The answers can be found on page 84.

1. $140 \div 7 =$ 2. $55 \div 5 =$

3. $72 \div 6 =$ 4. $120 \div 5 =$

5. $360 \div 9 =$ 6. $96 \div 8 =$

Self-assessment progress check

Multiplying decimals

The recap question below will help to consolidate your learning about multiplying with decimals. This question also involves a division. The answers can be found on page 84.

A patient has recently been admitted to the medical ward where you are working. During the admission process it was found that their body weight was 65.25 kilograms and the patient wants to know what this is in stones and pounds. One kilogram is the equivalent of 2.2 pounds, and there are 14 pounds to each stone. Convert the patient's weight from kilograms to stones and pounds.

Factors

When calculating using multiplication or division, you may have noticed some patterns in the numbers. A number like 32 can be broken down into **factors** that can be multiplied together to re-form 32. Factors of 32 include 4 and 8.

$32 \div 4 = 8$

and

$32 \div 8 = 4$

and

$4 \times 8 = 32$

When calculating, try to identify factors of numbers as this will help develop your skills in multiplication and division.

PERCENTAGES AND FRACTIONS

It is frequently necessary to break down numerical values into smaller units, or to make them easier to understand and more relevant. This is done without thought in everyday life but, as soon as links are made to maths or numeracy, there is a suspicion that this must be complicated. A phrase like 'eight out of ten cats prefer . . .' not only communicates the cat food manufacturer's name, but also gives a readily understandable statistic of consumer preference.

Percentages

The words 'per cent' are a common feature of everyday language, indicated by the symbol %. Nurses need an understanding of percentages and how to calculate them, as they are frequently used in nursing practice. In a patient who has sustained burns, the severity is partly calculated by estimating the amount of body surface affected, and is quoted as a percentage of the total body surface area. Percentages are used in the administration of medicines such as hydrocortisone cream. This is used in the management of skin disorders like eczema, and is available in strengths of 1% and 2.5%. Routine nursing observations require an understanding of percentages as the oxygen saturation level (SaO_2) of patients is quoted as a percentage, the normal range being 93–98% (Allibone and Nation, 2006). Most intravenous fluids have their contents indicated by percentages such as, for example, Dextrose 5%.

While percentages are commonly used in practice, an understanding of them is also valuable for academic study, because statistical information may be given in percentages. The Office for National Statistics (2006) advises of changes in household composition between 1971 and 2001. It reports an increase in the number of one-person households from 18% in 1971 to 29% in 2001, with the number staying at this level in 2005. Jukes and Gilchrist (2006) studied the numeracy skills of nursing students and reported an 82% response rate. They also found that nursing students did not have the ability to perform drug calculations at a 90% mastery level. Without an understanding of the meaning of percentages and how they are calculated, such information is of little use.

Calculating percentages

When calculating percentages, it is important to remember that the meaning of per cent is 'part of a hundred' and is written using the symbol %.

Example 1
A group of 132 student nurses have recently started their pre-registration training. There are 17 males and 115 females. What percentage of the group is female?

Method
The percentage is calculated by placing the number that we want to find the percentage for (115) over the total number in the group (132), this means dividing the top number by the bottom number. The answer to this is then multiplied by 100.

Process
Number female students = $\dfrac{115}{132} \times 100 = 87.12\%$ of group female
Total in group =

$\dfrac{17}{132} \times \dfrac{100}{1} = 12.88\%$ of the group is male.

Fractions

Fractions are an alternative to decimals when breaking down whole items into smaller units, or when quantifying numbers that are less than one. They can be viewed as part of a whole number, or one number divided by another. The reason why an understanding of fractions will be useful in clinical practice may not be immediately obvious, but this is possibly because fractions really are a part of our daily language like, for example, half an hour.

In nursing it is likely that the most common use of a fraction will be to quantify an amount that is less than one. A situation when this might occur is in the number of staff needed to run a hospital ward or department. A full-time nurse works $37\frac{1}{2}$ hours each week, which is one whole time equivalent. During the same week, a nurse who is half ($\frac{1}{2}$) of a whole-time equivalent will work 18 hours 45 minutes.

Fractions like $\frac{1}{2}$ are termed **proper fractions** and are the type of fractions that nurses are most likely to use. Proper fractions can be identified by the number above the line (1), called the **numerator**, being smaller than the number below the line (2), known as the **denominator**. The fraction $\frac{1}{2}$ means one part of two, where two is the whole. A fraction of $\frac{3}{5}$ means three parts of five, where five is the whole.

Improper fractions can be identified by the numerator being larger than the denominator. They can be converted into a mixed number. An example of an improper fraction is $\frac{7}{4}$ and this can be converted to $1\frac{3}{4}$. Improper fractions are rarely used in the clinical environment.

RATIOS

Sometimes it is necessary to provide a value that indicates a relationship or comparison between two items, or a **ratio**. In clinical practice, the drug epinephrine, used in the treatment of anaphylaxis and cardiac arrest, is available in several strengths, which are expressed in ratio form. Epinephrine is available in 1 millilitre ampoules with a ratio of 1 in 1 000, and 10 millilitre ampoules at 1 in 10 000. When related to drugs, the first number represents weight in grams and the second number represents volume in millilitres.

1 in 1 000 epinephrine equals 1 gram in 1 000 millilitres or, because each gram is the equivalent of 1 000 milligrams, there are 1 000 milligrams in 1 000 millilitres. This equates to 1 milligram in 1 millilitre, or 1 milligram per millilitre. 1 in 10 000 epinephrine equals 1 gram in 10 000 millilitres, and because each gram is the equivalent of 1 000 milligrams, there are 1 000 milligrams in 10 000 millilitres. This equates to 1 milligram in 10 millilitres.

The use of ratios is not confined to drug strengths. You will come across ratios when studying the frequency of a disease or disorder within a population, and you may see nurse-to-patient ratios quoted when reading about managing patient care.

EXPRESSING LARGE NUMBERS

Occasionally you may see numbers written in an exponential form. Exponential, or **power,** forms are ways of making very large or very small numbers more manageable by reducing the number of zeros. In clinical practice you are most likely to see this used on blood results from the laboratory or, perhaps, in a physiology book indicating the normal ranges of the cellular components of blood. For example, a neutrophil (a type of white cell) count can range between 2.0 and 7.5 $\times$ 10^9 per litre. The small raised nine next to the 10 tells you that 10 is being multiplied with itself nine times, effectively telling you how many times to move the decimal point.

So: 10^9 means $10 \times 10 \times 10 \times 10 \times 10 \times 10 \times 10 \times 10 \times 10$

SUMMARY
- Because of the complex numerical values used in the clinical environment, nurses need to be familiar with the decimal system and understand the role of the decimal point. This is a pre-requisite for working with SI units and calculating drug doses.
- Zeros play a vital role within a number, but can be a source of error if they act as trailing zeros.
- It is essential that nurses can calculate using the methods of addition, subtraction, multiplication and division as a basis for safe numeracy practice within the clinical environment.
- An understanding of percentages and ratios is fundamental to understanding the strength of some drugs.

Practice tip

While practice doesn't always guarantee perfection, it is the most important way of developing confidence and competence with calculations. Try to perform calculations longhand to revise the basics of arithmetic – don't cheat and resort to the calculator on your mobile phone.

FURTHER READING

BBC Bitesize maths
www.bbc.co.uk/schools/gcsebitesize/maths
The 'Number: intermediate and higher' section provides great revision on fractions, percentages, powers, ratios and proportions.

BBC Skillswise
www.bbc.co.uk/skillswise/numbers/wholenumbers
This website gives great tips and advice about the basics of calculating, plus information on ratios, factors, number and place values, as well as times table practice.

http://learntech.uwe.ac.uk/numeracy
This is a resource of a wide range of learning materials to help health care professionals improve their numeracy skills. Particularly relevant to this chapter are the sections on decimals, percentages and ratios. Contains some interactive tests.

Multiplication grid

0	1	2	3	4	5	6	7	8	9	10	11	12
1	1	2	3	4	5	6	7	8	9	10	11	12
2	2	4	6	8	10	12	14	16	18	20	22	24
3	3	6	9	12	15	18	21	24	27	30	33	36
4	4	8	12	16	20	24	28	32	36	40	44	48
5	5	10	15	20	25	30	35	40	45	50	55	60
6	6	12	18	24	30	36	42	48	54	60	66	72
7	7	14	21	28	35	42	49	56	63	70	77	84
8	8	16	24	32	40	48	56	64	72	80	88	96
9	9	18	27	36	45	54	63	72	81	90	99	108
10	10	20	30	40	50	60	70	80	90	100	110	120
11	11	22	33	44	55	66	77	88	99	110	121	132
12	12	24	36	48	60	72	84	96	108	120	132	144

Chapter 3

The SI System

INTRODUCTION

This chapter describes the SI system and the common units of measurement for weight and volume. Conventions for the use of SI unit abbreviations are discussed and ways of minimising the risk of confusion in clinical practice are considered. Non-SI units are also referred to where these are used clinically, as in the measurement of blood pressure. The recap self-testing material will allow practice to develop the ability and confidence to work with SI units.

THE SI SYSTEM

The SI system is an adaptation of the metric system and is almost universally employed in business, science and health care. The name SI is an abbreviation of the 'International System of Units', which was derived from the French 'le Système International d'Unités'.

There is a frequent need within clinical practice to express numerical values. This might include the urine output of a patient, the amount of a drug to be administered or the flow rate of an intravenous infusion. In addition to the numerical value, there is a need to specify a unit of measurement and a need for those units to be common across all health care environments, and also, ideally, in daily life. Using units of measurement that are familiar in everyday life should make the transition to becoming a nurse easier and safer than trying to learn a whole new system. It's likely that you already know most of the common units used in clinical practice. Volume is measured in **litres**, weight measured in **kilograms** and pressure measured in **millimetres of mercury**.

SI prefixes

SI units are used to quantify measurements, some extremely large and some extremely small. There are standard prefixes used to describe and name the quantities involved, irrespective of what is being measured. The most commonly used prefixes that apply to clinical practice are:

- **Mega** – this prefix indicates millions. Benzylpenicillin, a penicillin antibiotic that is administered by injection, is available in vials containing 600 **milligrams**. This is equivalent to one million international units, or one mega unit.
- **Milli** – this prefix indicates a thousandth of a unit. One milligram is one thousandth of a **gram**.
- **Micro** – this prefix indicates a millionth of a unit. One **microgram** is one millionth of a gram. (There are one thousand micrograms in one milligram and one thousand milligrams in one gram. One thousand multiplied by one thousand equals one million.)
- **Nano** – this prefix indicates a thousand-millionth of a unit. This is extremely small and rarely used in clinical practice.

SI Units

Volume

In clinical practice there is a need to measure very small amounts so there are smaller 'sub-units' of measurement. Litres are subdivided into millilitres, with 1 000 millilitres equal to one litre. The standard abbreviation for litre is L and the abbreviation for millilitres is ml. Within the SI system it is standard practice that unit abbreviations are written in the lower case but, because litre abbreviated to 'l' could be confused with the figure '1', it is the only unit abbreviated to a capital letter 'L'. It is also important to remember that when expressing plurals, there is no 's' on the end of the abbreviated form. We may talk of a patient passing 325 millilitres of urine but when this is written it becomes 325 ml. It is also standard practice that the abbreviated form of the SI unit does not have a full stop after it, unless it is at the end of a sentence.

The SI system has units smaller than millilitres for the measurement of volume. Millilitres can be subdivided into smaller units known as **microlitres**, with 1 000 microlitres in one millilitre. However, microlitres are rarely used in clinical practice.

Key point summary
1 litre (L) = 1 000 millilitres (ml)
1 ml = 0.001 L

Weight

The SI unit of weight is the kilogram, which can be subdivided into smaller units several times. Kilograms are useful when measuring large items like body weight but, when measuring small amounts of drugs, alternative units of measurement are needed. The unit smaller than one kilogram is a gram, and 1 000 grams equal one kilogram. The abbreviation for gram is g. Grams are used within clinical practice (for example, two paracetamol tablets are the equivalent of one gram) but it is frequently necessary to measure units much smaller than this.

Grams can be divided into smaller units called milligrams, with 1 000 milligrams, abbreviation mg, being the equivalent of one gram. Morphine is an opioid analgesic frequently used to control severe pain. It can be injected (intramuscularly, intravenously and subcutaneously) and administered orally. As an oral solution, it contains 10 mg in 5 ml.

Milligrams can also be divided into smaller units known as micrograms, with 1 000 micrograms being the equivalent of one milligram. There are two abbreviated forms of microgram, mcg and μ, but the use of these in clinical practice is controversial. For patient safety reasons, many hospitals demand that microgram is written in full to avoid confusion with mg. Digoxin is a cardiac glycoside used in heart failure and for some cardiac arrhythmias. The amount of drug taken daily could be 62.5 micrograms, 125 micrograms, 250 micrograms or even 500 micrograms. It is a commonly prescribed drug, with serious side effects should an overdose occur, so it is critical that the basic rules regarding abbreviations are observed.

Practice tip

Conventions for prescriptions state that drugs should be prescribed in whole amounts and not decimal fractions. In the case of digoxin this means that a prescription should read 125 micrograms, not 0.125 mg, so you must be able to convert between units. As a general rule:
- converting from a larger unit to a smaller unit means that you multiply by 1 000;
- converting from a smaller unit to a larger unit means that you divide by 1 000;
- converting from a larger unit to a smaller unit
  To convert 0.125 mg to micrograms
  0.125 × 1 000 = 125 micrograms

It's useful to remember that when multiplying by 1 000, the decimal point moves three places to the right. 0.125 becomes 125;

- converting from a smaller unit to a larger unit
  To convert 125 micrograms to milligrams
  125 ÷ 1 000 = 0.125 mg
Remember that when dividing by 1 000, the decimal point moves three places to the left. 125 becomes 0.125

Key point summary
1 000 micrograms (mcg) = 1 milligram (mg)
1 000 milligrams (mg) = 1 gram (g)
1 000 grams (g) = I kilogram (kg)

Practice tip
Care is still needed when measuring large amounts such as body weight. Two children received double the normal dose of medication in an X-ray department simply because their weight had been measured and recorded in pounds rather than kilograms (Department of Health, 2000).

Pressure

The commonly used unit for the measurement of blood pressure in clinical practice within the United Kingdom is millimetres of mercury, which has the abbreviation mmHg. You will see this displayed on sphygmomanometers used to measure and record a patient's blood pressure.

There is also an SI unit for pressure called the **pascal** (abbreviation Pa), which is named after the French physicist and mathematician Blaise Pascal (1623–62). The pascal is a small unit so you are more likely to see it referred to using the prefix **kilo**, as kilopascal (kPa). The prefix kilo means 1 000, so one kPa is equal to 1 000 pascals. One kPa is equal to approximately 7.5 mmHg (Woodrow, 2004). Unusually the abbreviated form of pascal has a capital letter; this is because it is named after someone.

It may seem a little confusing to have two units of measurement, but staff working in clinical practice do need to be aware of both. The kPa is recognised as the standard unit for measuring blood gases in the UK (Allibone and Nation, 2006), so you are likely to come across blood gas analysis reports using kPa in intensive care and high dependency units, and on respiratory wards. The use of the kPa isn't universal though and within some hospitals you will see mmHg used for blood gases.

Self-assessment progress check

SI units

In clinical practice it is essential that you understand the SI and other units used in the measurement of patient data, and you should be able to convert the various units used to measure volume and weight. The recap questions below will help to achieve this and the answers can be found on pages 84–86.

How many:
  1. Milligrams (mg) in a gram (g)?
  2. Micrograms (mcg) in a milligram (mg)?
  3. Milligrams (mg) in a kilogram (kg)?
  4. Millilitres (ml) in a litre (L)?
  5. Grams (g) in a kilogram (kg)?

Working between SI units. Convert:
  1. 1 200 mg into grams (g)
  2. 1.5 mg into micrograms (mcg)
  3. 2 kg into grams (g)
  4. 0.75 mg into micrograms (mcg)
  5. 625 ml into litres (L)
  6. 1 450 g into kilograms (kg)
  7. 0.728 L into millilitres (ml)
  8. 5 mg into grams (g)
  9. 0.05 mg into micrograms (mcg)
10. 0.0025 L into millilitres (ml)

Which is larger?
  1. 60 ml or 0.6 L?
  2. 1.1 mg or 1 010 mcg?
  3. 0.5 g or 750 mg?
  4. 0.4 mg or 40 mcg?
  5. 250 ml or 0.275 L?
  6. 25 g or 0.0025 kg?
  7. 75 mcg or 0.705 mg?
  8. 2 g or 0.2 mg?
  9. 0.045 L or 450 ml?
10. 25 mcg or 0.25 mg?

Add together the following amounts, expressing your answer in mg and micrograms.
  1. 30 micrograms (mcg) + 7 mg + 0.001 g =
  2. 0.25 mg + 1.06 mg + 0.004 g =

Add together the following amounts, expressing your answer in ml and L.

3. 0.1 L + 0.011 L + 0.605 L + 0.425 L =

Add together the following amounts.

4. A patient is prescribed 300 mg of a drug to be taken at breakfast and lunchtime, and a dose of 450 mg in the evening. Expressing your answers in milligrams and grams, what is the total amount of the drug taken each day?

5. A patient is advised not to exceed a daily salt intake of 6 g. If breakfast contained 1 400 mg, lunch 800 mg, dinner 2 000 mg and snacks and drinks throughout the day contained 600 mg, what is the total salt intake for a day? Express your answer in mg and g.

6. A patient takes three 30 mcg tablets daily. She plans to go on holiday and will need to take sufficient tablets for 14 days. Expressed in mg, how much of the drug will she take with her?

7. The local health centre is open Monday to Friday each week. The domestic mops the corridor floor and waiting area twice each day using 0.275 L of cleaning fluid each time. The cleaning fluid is supplied in containers that hold 4 500 ml. Expressed in ml and L, how much cleaning fluid will be left in the container at the end of the week?

8. A liquid medicine contains 20 mg in 5 ml
   a. How many mg are in 25 ml?
   b. How many mg are in 2.5 ml?
   c. How many mg are in 7.5 ml?

SUMMARY

- The SI system is designed to be a universal and comprehensive system of measurement units.
- The system is supported by a series of standardised prefixes that are common to all units of measurement. Once learned, these help to describe the size of the measurement.
- Measurements of volume, weight and pressure are common in clinical practice. Volume is usually measured in millilitres and litres, weight in micrograms, milligrams, grams and kilograms and pressure in kilopascals and millimetres of mercury.
- Recording patient data in non-SI units where it would normally be recorded in SI units can lead to serious errors when drug doses are calculated.

FURTHER READING

Useful as reference material, The National Physical Laboratory website at **www.npl.co.uk/reference** provides detailed information about SI units, prefixes and the conventions of the system.

A Dictionary of Units by Frank Tapson is available at **www.cleavebooks. co.uk/dictunit/dictunit1.htm**
This is an excellent dictionary of SI units, which covers prefixes, units and conventions. It also gives a history of the development of the system as well as including metric and imperial measurements used across the world.

Practice tip

There are some basic rules for calculating drug doses, which contribute to minimising the risk of error, irrespective of the route of administration.

- The prescribed dose and the available drug must be in the same unit of measurement, so convert if necessary.
- Use an equation and write down each step of the calculation.
- If you are performing a calculation that needs to be checked by another person, make sure you don't show them your answer or working out before they have arrived at an answer independently.
- If a calculation seems extremely complex, discuss this with the prescriber and a pharmacist. There may be a simpler way of arriving at the required dose.

Calculating for oral administration

Tablets and capsules

Some drug calculations appear quite straightforward, can be performed using a 'mental maths' approach and without the apparent need to use a written equation. For example, a patient is prescribed ampicillin 500 mg orally. The available **capsules** are 250 mg, so there is a need to administer two capsules because $250 \times 2 = 500$. Even though the calculation doesn't require any complicated arithmetic, it is important to understand how you arrived at the answer. This type of calculation is used quite often when administering liquid medicines and can also be useful for some injections. Although multiplication was used in the calculation, there is also a pattern of ratios: one capsule equals 250 mg, two capsules equal 500 mg, three capsules equal 750 mg, four capsules equal 1 000 mg (1 g) and so on.

Practice tip

When calculating tablets it is possible that your answer could indicate the need to give half a tablet. Remember, only tablets that are scored should be cut as not all tablets are suitable for splitting in half. Ideally the correct-strength tablet should be administered. Capsules are not suitable for splitting and very small tablets cannot be split in half accurately. Any tablets with a specialised coating such as **enteric coating**, which is designed to delay the breakdown of the drug, must not be split. Cutting an enteric-coated tablet could cause serious harm to a patient.

With nurses spending up to 40% of their day administering medicines (Audit Commission, 2001), calculating the number of tablets or capsules to administer is a frequent event. Try the recap questions below to help become familiar and competent in this. The answers can be found on pages 86–87.

Self-assessment progress check

Calculating tablets

1. A patient is prescribed 5 mg of bendroflumethiazide. How many 2.5 mg tablets should be given?
2. A patient is prescribed 7.5 mg of soluble prednisolone orally. How many 5 mg tablets should be given?
3. A patient is prescribed 120 mg of furosemide. How many 40 mg tablets should be given?
4. A patient is prescribed 250 mcg of digoxin. How many 125 mcg tablets should be given?
5. A patient is prescribed 40 mg of gliclazide. How many 80 mg tablets should be given?

Liquid medicines

The ratio-type equation used to calculate the number of tablets to administer can also be used for liquid medicines to be given orally. It can be used to find out how many milligrams of the drug are contained in each millilitre of the solution.

Example 1: A patient is prescribed morphine solution (Oramorph®) 8 mg. The solution contains 10 mg in 5 ml. To find out how many mg per ml there are in the solution: divide the 10 (mg) by 5 (ml), $10 \div 5 = 2$, so each ml of solution contains 2 mg of morphine. The required dose is 8 mg, so it is necessary to administer 4 ml of morphine solution because 4 (ml) × 2 (mg) = 8 mg.

There are occasions when an alternative approach is needed, such as when the prescribed dose is smaller or larger than the standard preparation. There are several versions of the equation that can be used, but one of the most commonly applied ones is known as the 'WIG' equation. 'WIG' stands for 'Want, In, Got'. The WIG equation is

$$\frac{\text{What you } \mathbf{WANT} \times \text{What it is } \mathbf{IN}}{\text{What you have } \mathbf{GOT}}$$

This equation instructs you to multiply the required drug dose (want) by the amount it is in (in), and then divide this by the strength of the drug available (got).

Example 2: A patient is prescribed diazepam **elixir** 10 mg. The label indicates that the stock available contains 5 mg in 5 ml. To calculate the volume of elixir to be administered use the WIG equation. Applying the rules for calculating drug doses means that the drug must be in the same units. In this example they are – both the prescribed dose and the elixir are in milligrams – so no conversion is necessary. The equation can now be written as:

$$\frac{10 \times 5}{5} = \frac{50}{5} = 10 \text{ ml of diazepam elixir should be given to the patient}$$

Example 3: A patient is prescribed 1 g of metformin syrup. The label indicates that the stock available contains 500 mg in 5 ml. To calculate the volume of elixir to be administered use the WIG equation. Applying the rules for calculating drug doses means that the drug must be in the same units. In this example the prescribed dose is in grams but the syrup is labelled in milligrams so it is necessary to convert both into the same units. The units need to be converted to the smaller unit so that the equation involves whole numbers rather than decimal fractions. As 1 g is equivalent to 1 000 mg, this will be put into the equation:

What you **Want** = 1 000
What it is **In** = 5
What you have **Got** = 500

The equation can now be written as:

$$\frac{1\,000 \times 5}{500} = \frac{5\,000}{500} = 10 \text{ ml of metformin syrup should be given to the patient}$$

Try the recap questions below before moving onto the calculating injections section. The answers can be found on page 87.

Self-assessment progress check

Calculating oral liquids

1. An adult is prescribed 300 mg of sodium valproate oral solution. The bottle label states there are 200 mg in 5 ml. What volume of sodium valproate needs to be administered?

2. A child is prescribed 12 mg of furosemide oral solution. The bottle label states there are 8 mg per ml. What volume of sodium furosemide needs to be administered?

3. A child is prescribed 62.5 mg of phenoxymethylpenicillin (Penicillin V) oral solution. The bottle label states there are 125 mg in 5 ml. What volume of phenoxymethylpenicillin needs to be administered?

4. A patient is prescribed 210 mg of ferrous fumarate syrup. The bottle label states there are 140 mg in 5 ml. What volume of ferrous fumarate needs to be administered?

5. An adult is prescribed 250 mg of amoxicillin oral suspension. The bottle label states there are 125 mg in 5 ml. What volume of amoxicillin needs to be administered?

Practice tip

Numeracy and calculation skills will help to reduce errors when performing calculations, but they can also help you to select the correct preparation when reading medicine container labels. This is why an understanding of SI units is an integral part of performing safe calculations. For example, morphine is a commonly prescribed opiate drug with a **narrow therapeutic range**. Overdose can lead to respiratory depression and hypotension. It can be administered orally, rectally or by injection and, in oral immediate-release form, it is available in five different strengths ranging from 10 to 100 mg. In a controlled-release form, oral morphine is available in 12 different strengths from 5 to 200 mg. Clearly, the ability to read and understand the strength of a drug is essential to safe calculation.

Calculating for administration by injection

Example 1: A patient is prescribed hydrocortisone 40 mg as an intramuscular injection. Ampoules containing 50 mg in 2 ml are available. Calculate the volume required for the injection.

Use the WIG equation: $\dfrac{\text{What you WANT} \times \text{What it is IN}}{\text{What you have GOT}}$

and insert the details of this calculation giving:

$$\frac{40 \times 2}{50} = \frac{80}{50} = 1.6 \text{ ml}$$

or drugs are being administered. In these situations it is necessary to be able to calculate the number of drops per minute required to infuse the fluid over the prescribed time.

Administration sets vary but, generally, a standard intravenous administration set has 20 drops per ml and a blood administration set has 15 drops per ml.

To calculate the number of drops per minute, the amount of fluid to be infused needs to be converted from litres to millilitres and then put into the following equation:

$$\frac{\text{Volume prescribed (ml)}}{\text{Hours of infusion}} \times \frac{\text{Drops per ml of administration set}}{60 \text{ minutes}}$$

Example 1: 500 ml of Sodium Chloride 0.9% is prescribed as an intravenous infusion over 4 hours. Inserting these figures into the equation gives:

$$\frac{500}{4} \times \frac{20}{60} = 125 \times 0.33 \text{ (recurring)} = 41.25$$

but 41 drops per minute are used to avoid over infusion, and to prevent air entering the infusion administration set.

Precision of measurement

The results of some calculations need to be expressed with extreme precision but, with many everyday calculations, this is unnecessary and could cause confusion. There are very few clinical calculations that need to be expressed beyond two decimal places, i.e. the digits appearing to the right of the decimal point. For example, the distance from a local district general hospital to the nearest community hospital is accepted as 15 miles. In reality, the distance could be 15 miles 192.5 yards. The extra information communicated in the precise answer serves no useful purpose.

Similarly, when calculating how fast an intravenous infusion should flow, digits to the right of the decimal point are of little value because they are less than one drop and therefore can't be administered. There is a general principle about 'rounding off' numbers where a high degree of precision isn't required – numbers including five or more round up and numbers including four or less round down. Therefore, the number 9.57 correct to one decimal place is rounded up to 9.6. The digit '7' in the second decimal place is equal to or greater than five, so rounds up making the digit '5' in the first decimal place into a '6'. Similarly, 9.54 correct to one decimal place becomes 9.5 because the digit '4' in the second decimal place is equal to four or less and therefore rounds down, resulting in 9.5.

When performing drops per minute calculations for intravenous infusions, it may seem like the rounding-off principle is being used, but it isn't. It is always sensible to round down to avoid completely emptying the bag of fluid, causing air to enter the infusion-giving set tubing.

Administering intravenous infusions without the control of a volumetric pump isn't an exact science as there are other factors that influence the rate of administration. The position of the limb and height of the fluid above the intravenous **cannula** both play a role in the flow rate. This means that calculating the number of drops per minute necessary to infuse fluids over a specific period of time isn't highly precise, but it is far more accurate than an estimate.

Sometimes, when calculating flow rates, the result involves a recurring number. For example, 1 000 ml of fluid given intravenously over 6 hours means that 166.6666666 ml / hour need to be infused. Mathematically, this could be rounded up to 167 ml / hour but in clinical practice could result in an empty infusion bag and air entering the administration set.

The questions below should help you to become more familiar with calculating drops per minute. Check your answers with those on pages 90–91.

Self-assessment progress check

Intravenous infusion drop rates

1. A patient is prescribed 1 000 ml of intravenous Sodium Chloride 0.9% to run over 6 hours. Using a standard intravenous infusion set, how many drops per minute are needed to infuse the fluid over the prescribed time?
2. A patient is prescribed 500 ml of intravenous Dextrose 5% to run over 4 hours. Using a standard intravenous infusion set, how many drops per minute are needed to infuse the fluid over the prescribed time?
3. A patient is prescribed 1 000 ml of intravenous Ringer's solution to run over 8 hours. Using a standard intravenous infusion set, how many drops per minute are needed to infuse the fluid over the prescribed time?
4. A patient is prescribed 500 ml of intravenous Sodium Chloride 0.9% to run over 6 hours. Using a standard intravenous infusion set, how many drops per minute are needed to infuse the fluid over the prescribed time?

Example 1: A patient is prescribed 15 units of heparin (unfractioned) per kilogram of body weight per hour. The patient weighs 45 kg so the equation is:

$15 \times 45 = 675$ units per hour

Over a 24-hour period this will mean that 16 200 units of heparin will be administered.

Example 2: A patient is prescribed epinephrine (adrenaline) 0.2 micrograms per kilogram of body weight per minute. The patient weighs 90 kg so the equation is:

$0.2 \times 90 = 18$ mcg per minute

Drugs prescribed to be administered intravenously per minute will be diluted into an appropriate intravenous fluid. Depending on the dilution of the drug there will also be a 'rate of infusion' type calculation to be performed. The drugs used in the two examples above require a high degree of control during infusion and would therefore be given via a volumetric pump or syringe driver. However, there is still a need to be able to calculate the volume to be infused to check that the pump or syringe driver is working correctly.

In the future it is hoped that information technology systems will play a role in reducing the number of errors made when administering drugs (Department of Health, 2004a), but an absolutely foolproof system is a long way off and is probably impossible to develop. Information technology developments like computerised prescribing with decision support, or bar coding of medication administration records and drugs, are likely to be introduced as and when the technology is available, proven and affordable. Gradual changes in technological support will mean that individual health professionals will still require the same calculation skills and knowledge about the units used to measure drugs as they do now. Indeed, health professionals are warned about becoming too dependent on computerised systems and automated solutions. There are already examples of patients receiving the wrong doses of radiotherapy and chemotherapy that have been recommended by an automated system, yet the errors have not been recognised by staff.

SUMMARY
- Accurately calculating a drug dose is only one of several complex stages in the safe administration of medicines.
- In your eagerness to perform any calculations correctly, don't neglect the use of a safe checking procedure to ensure the drug is

---

administered to the right patient.
- Drug calculations require more than arithmetical skills. It is important to be aware of the circumstances that have contributed to calculation errors in the past.
- Although volumetric pumps calculate the rate of infusion for you, don't neglect to use your calculation skills to check this.
- Some drug calculations are fairly complex. Use an equation to help break each calculation into stages.

FURTHER READING

Haigh, S. (2002) 'How to calculate drug dosage accurately: advice for nurses'. *Professional Nurse*, 18(1): 54–7
This article, written by a pharmacist, contains the basic calculation equations and applies them to a wide variety of examples. It also contains a short quiz to test your understanding.

Higgins, D. (2005) 'Drug calculations'. *Nursing Times*, 101(46): 24–5
This is a very short but useful overview from a senior critical care nurse. It covers the basics about calculating dosages as well as including conversions between SI units. It is valuable as an introduction or to revise and refresh previous learning.

Trim, J. (2004) 'Clinical skills: a practical guide to working out drug calculations'. *British Journal of Nursing*, 13(10): 602–6
A good all-round review of the essentials of calculating dosages, which is well applied to practice. It also considers some of the professional issues like why mistakes happen and how to reduce errors.

www.testandcalc.com/drugcalc/index.asp
This web-based American resource provides a useful range of information and quizzes about drug calculations. There is the option to subscribe for additional learning materials and support, but the freely accessible parts are interactive, colourful and educational.

www.lanpdc.scot.nhs.uk/calculations/dc.asp
This web resource from Lanarkshire in Scotland provides the opportunity to test your drug calculation ability in a wide range of situations. The site offers clues and help with the calculation, as well as including an on-screen calculator.

Chapter 5

Clinical Calculations

INTRODUCTION

Concerns about the numeracy skills of health care professionals are often linked to doubts about the performance of drug calculations and the safe administration of medicines. There are many situations where numeracy skills are required in daily clinical work, and the consequences of errors have the same potential for harm as a drug calculation mistake. This chapter explores some of the risk assessment tools used in clinical practice and discusses factors that influence their accuracy. The need to have a working knowledge of the **pH scale** is discussed and the chapter shows that this is a prerequisite for the safe performance of some clinical skills. Other commonly performed clinical calculations are also discussed, including fluid balance measurement and nutritional screening, in order to emphasise that other professional skills in addition to numeracy are required to ensure accuracy.

NUMERACY SKILLS IN CLINICAL PRACTICE

In nursing there seems to be a natural tendency to associate numeracy skills only with drug calculations. This is an understandable link because of the potential consequences of drug errors. Chapter Four explored some of the issues that contribute to drug calculation errors and stressed that numeracy skills are an essential component of many aspects of clinical practice. Errors in the measurement of numerical patient data like body weight or in the recording of numerical data using the wrong units may have similar consequences to the administration of a wrong drug dose.

The recently published Essential Skills Clusters (NMC, 2007a), which apply to all student nurses who commence training after September 2008, guide the clinical experience of student nurses and indicate which parts of practice depend on numeracy skills and will therefore require assessment in future. The Essential Skills Clusters indicate that modern clinical practice demands numerate practitioners, but also make it quite clear that, when applied to nursing, there is more to numeracy than drug calculations. In addition to the management of medicines, the Essential Skills Clusters indicate that numeracy skills are required for:

- the organisation of care and, specifically, the measurement, documentation and interpretation of vital signs;
- nutrition and fluid management, ensuring that patients receive adequate nutritional and fluid intake by assessing and monitoring nutritional and fluid status.

Students will need to demonstrate competence in these areas of practice before being eligible to join the register of nurses.

Patient assessment

Patient assessment involves the collection and analysis of a broad range of patient data, some in a numerical form. The assessment process uses **clinical risk assessment calculators** or tools to obtain patient data. There are claims that the risk of developing a pressure ulcer, malnutrition, sustaining a fall or requiring high-dependency care can be predicted by using an appropriate risk assessment calculator.

Sensitivity

With the possible exception of some aspects of nutritional assessment, the arithmetic involved in the use of clinical risk assessment calculators is usually confined to addition and subtraction. The calculations may seem straightforward but there are some complex issues to be considered when using such tools. These may not appear to be involved in the calculation of risk, but do need to be considered as they influence the accuracy of the tools. Clinical risk assessment calculators involve the collection of data and should be viewed with the same level of scrutiny as if they were being used in a research study. One measurement of the accuracy of a tool is sensitivity. This measures the extent to which the tool can identify the condition being examined in a sample of people who have the condition. It is the ratio of the number of people testing positive using the tool to the entire sample. Risk assessment calculators do not measure the presence of a condition as they are trying to establish the individual's risk of developing the condition. This is addressed by the tool containing indicators designed to identify patients who will go on to develop, for example, a pressure ulcer or sustain a fall. To be of any real value in clinical practice, an ideal tool would only indicate the patients at risk of developing the condition, as this would enable care and resources to be focused on those most in need. From this, you can see how critical it is that the tools only contain valid indicators.

Specificity

Another test of the accuracy of clinical risk assessment calculators is the specificity. Using the example of a falls risk calculator, the specificity measures how many patients did not sustain a fall, having been identified as of 'low risk' by the tool. The concepts of sensitivity and specificity may seem quite daunting, but if it is important to identify a patient's risk of developing serious and costly problems like pressure ulcers or falls, it makes sense to assess the risk as accurately as possible.

The accuracy and value of pressure ulcer risk assessment tools

Since the development of the Norton score in 1975 (Norton, Mclaren and Exton-Smith, 1975), there have been several pressure ulcer risk assessment tools designed with the intention of accurately identifying patients most at risk. Guidelines produced by NICE (2003) suggest that a pressure ulcer risk assessment calculator should be used as an *aide-mémoire*, but don't identify or recommend a specific tool. Tools need to be 'predictive, sensitive, specific, reliable, easy and convenient to use' (Wick, 2006 in Stephen-Haynes, 2006, p. 52), but many nurses doubt the accuracy and value of them (Thompson, 2005). Pancorbo-Hidalgo *et al.* (2006) systematically reviewed the effectiveness of risk assessment scales for pressure ulcer prevention and concluded that there was no evidence to suggest that the use of these tools decreased the incidence of pressure ulcers. They did identify both the Braden and Norton scales as being more accurate predictors of pressure ulcers than the clinical judgement of nurses.

Young (2004) draws attention to an important feature of the NICE guidelines. She highlights a change in the terminology used to describe the risk of developing pressure ulcers. Risk has traditionally been considered as 'low', 'medium', 'high' or 'very high', but this is replaced with 'vulnerable to pressure damage' for patients at low, medium and high levels of risk. Patients who were previously identified as being 'very high' risk are now considered as 'at an elevated risk of pressure ulcers'. The reason for this change is numeracy-based. If you look carefully at risk assessment scales, it soon becomes clear why these aren't perfect at identifying exactly which patients are at the highest or lowest risk of developing pressure ulcers. The Norton scale is one of many possible examples, as well as being the oldest pressure ulcer risk assessment scale. The original scale included the categories: general physical condition, mental state, activity, mobility and incontinence, though there have been additions to these over the years. Each of these categories is scored on a four-point scale giving a minimum overall score of 5 and a maximum of 20. It was initially considered that overall scores lower than 12 would inevitably lead to pressure ulcer development. What this and other clinical risk assessment scales do is to use a descriptor of a condition and assign a number to it. For example, the category of mobility:

- Full = 4
- Slightly limited = 3
- Very limited = 2
- Immobile = 1

There is order in the descriptors as they increase from 'immobile' to 'full', which is accompanied by an increase in the numerical score. The scores need to be viewed with caution because the difference between each descriptor within the category is not the same, but the numerical difference between 1 and 2, and 2 and 3 is exactly the same. The clinical risk assessment calculator uses the sum of several categories and has clearly defined numerical cut-off points to identify risk. A score lower than 12 is classed as at risk, yet scores above this are classed as being of low or no risk. It is easy to criticise clinical risk assessment tools because they fail to tell us exactly which patients are at what level of risk. This is a little unfair on the calculators and a little naïve to expect this. We may think that the tools are precise but, because of the way they measure indicators of risk, they simply can't be. Chapter Six explores this issue in more detail under 'levels of measurement'.

Key point summary
Clinical risk assessment calculators are intended to help staff identify patients at risk of developing serious problems such as pressure ulcers or sustaining a fall. The calculations involved are not too taxing, but the accuracy of these tools can be limited by design faults. This isn't a reason not to use them but it is a reason to use other sources of patient data as well.

The Modified Early Warning System

The Modified Early Warning System (MEWS) is a bedside clinical assessment tool used on admission units and general wards. It is designed to detect physiological deterioration in acutely ill patients by scoring observations of their vital signs (Palmer, 2004). The rationale for calculating a MEWS score is that there are limits on the number of patients who can occupy critical care beds at any one time. Identifying those who would most benefit from this resource seems a logical step, and the MEWS score is a method of achieving this. There is evidence that abnormal physiological measurements have been recorded on patients in the hours prior to cardiopulmonary arrest (Goldhill et al., 1999). This may be due to a lack

tubes being mistakenly inserted into the lung rather than the stomach, leading to the deaths of at least 11 patients between December 2002 and December 2004. The methods used to check the placement of feeding tubes have been found to be inaccurate (National Patient Safety Agency, 2005), which resulted in the advice to use pH paper to measure the acidity of gastric aspirate, rather than rely on litmus paper which only indicates whether the solution is an acid or alkaline. It is recommended that aspirate needs to be measured at pH 5.5 or below to confirm correct positioning. Blue litmus paper turns red when in contact with an acid, but Metheny *et al.* (1990) reported slightly acidic readings from the tracheo-bronchial tree of patients, which could lead to feeding commencing while the tube is positioned in the respiratory tract. Unfortunately, the National Patient Safety Agency (2007a) continues to report deaths and near misses because of feeding tube misplacement. A Europe-wide survey of adult intensive care units in 2007 found that the most commonly used test to establish correct feeding tube placement was the auscultatory method, reported by 72.6% of units (Fulbrook, Bongers and Albarran, 2007). This involves the injection of air down the tube while using a stethoscope to listen for bubbling or a 'whooshing' sound. However, advice from the National Patient Safety Agency (2005) clearly states that this method should not be used.

Key point summary
Understanding pH is necessary for routine care interventions like urine testing. It is also needed for patient safety when ascertaining that a feeding tube is in the correct position, prior to commencing a feed.

NUTRITIONAL STATUS

Nurses and midwives working in any clinical setting need to be aware that adequate nutrition is a prerequisite for the health and well-being of all patients, and that good nutrition plays a vital role in recovery from illness.

In 1859 Florence Nightingale commented that 'Every careful observer of the sick will agree in this that thousands of patients are annually starved in the midst of plenty', yet 135 years later McWhirter and Pennington (1994) reported the incidence of malnutrition in hospital as 40%. More than a decade later, there are still a significant number of issues that require addressing before nurses can claim to provide comprehensive nutritional care (Lecko, 2006).

Hydration

There are various nutrients required by the body including proteins, fats, carbohydrates, fibre, vitamins, minerals and water. Water is the most common molecule in the body and plays a key role as the most abundant solvent carrying other nutrients and waste. It is also involved in the regulation of body temperature. Water accounts for approximately 60% of the body weight of an adult male but this varies in women and children from 50% to 70%, depending on the amount of body fat. Factors that influence body fat, such as gender and diet, will also influence the total volume of body water. Those individuals with lower levels of body fat, like children, will have a higher volume of body water, and individuals with larger amounts of body fat, like women or those who are obese, will have a lower volume of water (Montague, Watson and Herbert, 2005). When calculating a patient's fluid balance, it is important to appreciate that individuals do vary. The calculations that you perform need to be accurate but don't lose sight of your patient; numbers might be standardised, but patients are unique.

The measurement of fluid input and output is common practice in many clinical settings. It is essential to remember the reasons for monitoring a patient's fluid balance to help ensure that it is performed accurately and is not treated as routine. Calculating fluid balance is part of the assessment of a patient's state of hydration, helping to identify those patients who are dehydrated and those who are at risk of dehydration (Holman, Roberts and Nicol, 2005). In healthy individuals and where patients are able to drink freely, the amount of fluid consumed is equal to the amount of fluid lost by the body. In adults, two to three litres of fluid intake daily are considered adequate. Excess water, wastes and electrolytes are excreted through the kidneys and in the faeces, with some water and salt loss via the skin and respiratory tract.

Inadequate hydration has been identified as a patient safety issue that can be a common problem in hospitals (National Patient Safety Agency, 2007b). This can rapidly lead to dehydration, a state where the loss of water from the body exceeds intake. If dehydration is not corrected, various physiological compensatory mechanisms maintain blood circulation but, if fluid depletion continues, blood pressure falls, pulse volume weakens and the heart rate rises. Ultimately this can result in renal failure and death.

There are many reasons why it becomes necessary to measure and record the fluid intake and output of patients and these generally fall into three categories. Firstly, there are situations where there is a problem with getting fluids into the body, like, for example, patients who have difficulties in swallowing. Secondly, there are situations where there may be disruption in the balance of water between the various compartments within the body, like, for example, a patient with hypovolaemic shock. Thirdly, there are situations where there are problems with excreting fluid from the body, as in patients with renal failure. These categories are not mutually exclusive and can exist together, as in the example of a patient with severe hypovolaemic shock who develops acute renal failure.

Practice tip
The ability to calculate fluid input and output is important, but calculations will only have value if records are complete. Poor fluid balance record keeping may result in the failure to identify patients who are dehydrated (Nutrition Now Campaign, 2007) and inaccurate recording will affect the validity of any calculations performed (Bryant, 2007). Make sure that the quality of your record keeping provides information that will contribute to accurate calculations and safe clinical practice.

Possible errors when calculating fluid balance

In Chapter Four, contextual factors that predisposed to calculation errors were explored. Although these were related to drug calculations, there are similar factors that will influence the accuracy of fluid balance calculations. These include increased amounts of **insensible loss**, difficulties in estimating the exact amount that a patient has drunk having left half a cup of tea, and judging urine output when a patient has suffered from urinary incontinence. When calculating the fluid intake and output of a patient, don't forget to use non-numerical information, as this may validate your calculations. Remember that close relatives may know the patient best and might have noticed changes. Checking the brightness of the eyes, observing if they appear sunken, and noting the smell of a patient's breath can be used to assess for dehydration. The colour of your patient's urine usually gives an indication of the concentration. Darker urine indicates that it is more concentrated and paler urine more dilute. This can be used as evidence of the quality of hydration. Calculations are useful, but don't neglect to consider the large amount of non-numerical data that is readily available in the clinical environment.

Fluid balance charts

Fluid balance charts can be a useful record of fluid intake and output, but the accuracy does depend on the staff using them. Different members of staff may interpret and record fluid intake or output differently. For example, do all staff record the volume of liquid foods like custard or soup on the chart? In many areas of practice, it is reasonable to think of fluid balance estimation rather than accurate measurement, with one or two exceptions like neonatal, paediatric and burns units.

The numeracy skills required to accurately complete fluid balance charts are addition, subtraction and possibly multiplication. While these are some of the basic number skills, it doesn't automatically follow that calculating fluid balance charts is easy. There are normally many small calculations to be performed and a lapse of concentration at a critical point may mean starting the calculation all over again or could lead to an error. Some charts help prevent this by having a 'running total' column.

Fluid balance charts are used to record all fluid intake and output over a 24-hour period, irrespective of the route of administration. Fluid loss from urine, diarrhoea, a stoma, wound drain or nasogastric tube aspirate is also recorded. At the end of the 24-hour period the total fluid intake and output is calculated, and an overall balance arrived at. If the amount of fluid taken into the body is greater than the amount lost from the body, this is called a positive fluid balance. If the loss is greater than intake, it is considered a negative fluid balance. A positive fluid balance might be found when a patient has been admitted in a dehydrated state and the body is replacing the fluid depletion. A negative fluid balance could be found in a patient with heart failure and **oedema** who has been given diuretic drugs. The excess fluid that has accumulated in the interstitial space is lost from the body, under the influence of the diuretic drugs.

Activity

Using the data supplied on the fluid balance chart (Figure 2), calculate the following:
1. the total oral intake;
2. the total intravenous intake;
3. the total fluid intake;
4. the total urine output;
5. the total fluid output;
6. the fluid balance for this 24-hour period, indicating whether this is positive or negative.

(The answers can be found on page 93.)

Fluid balance chart
Title:
Surname:
First name:
Patient / id number:
Ward / department:
Date:

	Intake			Output		
Time	Oral	Intravenous	Nasogastric Tube	Urine	Vomit / Aspirate	Drain
0600		100 ml Normal saline				
0700	Tea 150 ml			450 ml		
0800	Tea 150 ml					
0900	Fresh orange 100 ml					
1000	Coffee 150 ml			350 ml		
1100	Water 75 ml					
1200	Water 150 ml	100 ml Normal saline		375 ml		
1300	Tea 150 ml					50 ml
1400	Tea 150 ml					
1500	Water 75 ml			425 ml		
1600	Tea 150ml					
1700	Orange juice 150 ml					
1800	Water 100 ml	100 ml Normal saline		380 ml		
1900	Tea 150 ml					
2000	Chocolate 150 ml					
2200	Water 100 ml			450 ml		
2400		100 ml Normal saline				
24-hour Totals						

Figure 2 Fluid balance chart

Key point summary
- Just because the calculation of fluid input and output is commonly performed in clinical areas, don't treat it as routine. Remember there are good reasons for monitoring fluid balance and most of these relate to patient safety and well-being.
- Errors and omissions in the measurement and recording of fluid intake and output influence the accuracy of calculations.
- Don't ignore non-numerical patient data when assessing the state of a patient's hydration.

Nutrition

One of the fundamental roles of nurses when providing nutritional care is to identify patients most at risk of malnutrition by using a screening tool (McAtear, 2006). The aim of nutritional screening is to identify those most at risk of, or suffering from, malnutrition as well as to monitor the progress of patients already identified as being at risk. Patients with chronic diseases, the elderly or those recently discharged from hospital are most at risk (Elia, 2003), although it is worth remembering that malnutrition can affect anyone. There are challenges in assessing and monitoring the nutritional status of patients, ranging from a lack of scales needed to weigh patients, to the interruption of mealtimes by other clinical activities and, possibly, the lowly status afforded to nutritional care (Lecko, 2006).

The MUST tool

A recent audit of surgical and medical patients in a Scottish hospital revealed that only 26% of patients were routinely nutritionally screened on admission (Bell, 2007). Bell (2007) recommended that the 'Malnutrition Universal Screening Tool' (MUST) should be introduced (see Figure 3). The MUST screening tool is a valid measure of malnutrition in adults and is suitable for use across many clinical settings (McAtear, 2006). It is designed to be used by different health care professionals (Malnutrition Advisory Group, 2003a). There are many other published nutritional screening tools but, in some cases, there is a lack of evidence to support their use and many have not had their reliability and validity established (Malnutrition Advisory Group, 2003a). The appeal of the MUST screening tool is that it addresses these weaknesses and is designed to be universal. There are five steps in the application of the MUST tool:

1. the measurement of height and weight to calculate a body mass index (BMI);
2. identifying and calculating unplanned weight loss;
3. establishing the effect of acute disease;
4. the addition of the individual scores and calculation of the overall risk of malnutrition;
5. the planning and implementation of care to meet identified deficits.

The application of the MUST tool is supported by a comprehensive guide and explanatory booklet, which can be accessed at **www.bapen.org.uk**. The screening tool provides a BMI chart as well as details used to calculate a weight loss score. Apart from the value of these in calculating a MUST score, the charts are also useful for the conversion of metric measurements

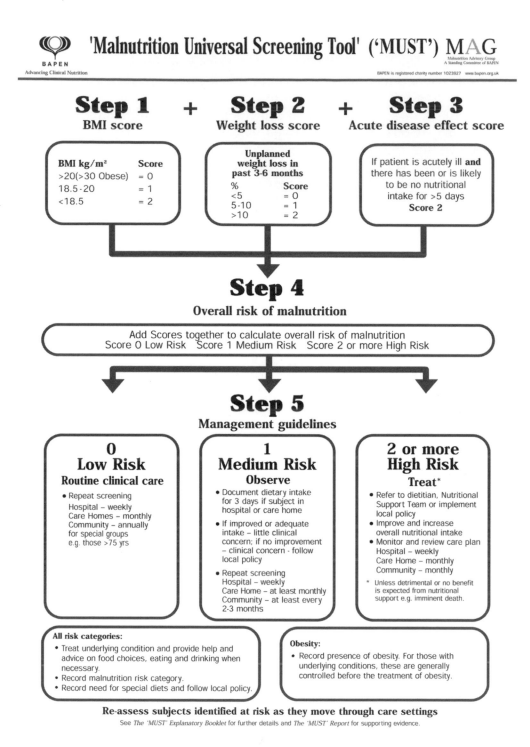

Figure 3 The five steps in the Malnutrition Universal Screening Tool (MUST). A comprehensive guide and explanatory booklet can be found at www.bapen.org.uk/must_tool.html. Reproduced with permission

for weight and height into imperial measures. In clinical calculations, metres and kilograms should be used, but many patients still want to know their height in feet and inches and weight in stones and pounds.

The first two steps in calculating a MUST score involve some measurements and calculations, but the BMI and weight loss data sheets included in the MUST pack reduce the need for anything too complex. However, there will be occasions when it is necessary to calculate these, possibly in clinical environments where the MUST tool has not been adopted.

Example 1
Calculating a BMI
The BMI is a reliable measure of the relationship between weight and height in adults, although it should be used with caution in older adults as it is not sensitive to the loss of height and muscle mass that can occur with advancing age (Johnstone, Farley and Hendry, 2006). The equation used to calculate a BMI is:

$$BMI = \frac{Weight\ (kg)}{Height\ (m^2)}$$

The unit of measurement for a BMI is kg/m^2, although this is frequently omitted and the BMI stated as a figure. If a patient weighed 73 kg and was 1.68 m tall, the BMI would be calculated as:

$$\frac{73}{1.68 \times 1.68} = \frac{73}{2.8224} = 25.86,\ \text{which is rounded up to 26 kg/m}^2$$

Using the BMI table below, a BMI of 26 puts the patient in the 'overweight' category.

BMI (kg/m²)	Weight status
Below 18.5	Underweight
18.5–24.9	Normal
25–29.9	Overweight
30–39.9	Obese
Above 40	Very obese
	(World Health Organization, 2005)

There are situations where it is impossible for patients to stand, or even get out of bed, and there is no recent reliable record of their weight. In these circumstances there are alternative methods of estimating a BMI. The 'Mid upper arm circumference' (MUAC), measured in centimetres, is recommended as an option. This involves the measurement around the

Self-assessment progress check

Ideal body weight calculations

The answers can be found on page 94.

Calculate the ideal body weight for the following:
1. A female who is 1.6 m (5 feet 3 inches) tall.
2. A male who is 1.78 m (5 feet 10 inches) tall.
3. A female who is 1.68 m (5 feet 6 inches) tall.
4. A male who is 1.7 m (5 feet 7 inches) tall.

SUMMARY

- In clinical practice there is more to numeracy skills than the calculation of drug doses. Numeracy is required for many aspects of patient care including the measurement of vital signs, assessing risk and monitoring nutritional and hydration status.
- The calculations performed when identifying 'at risk' scores using risk assessment tools are not overly complicated, but there are design factors that influence the accuracy of these tools and limit their usefulness.
- Although pH may seem complicated, an understanding of it will help you to grasp the physiological changes that can occur in some seriously ill patients and appreciate the rationale for some clinical procedures.
- Inadequate hydration is a threat to patient safety and measuring fluid intake and output is vital to the well-being of many patients. Accuracy depends on the ability to calculate as well as agreement and consistency of measurement between different staff, and the quality of record keeping.
- Malnutrition continues to be part of modern health care and yet there are reliable and valid ways of measuring and monitoring nutritional status. The MUST score offers health care staff a risk assessment calculator which can be used in many clinical environments to identify patients at risk, as well as recommending additional care.

FURTHER READING

Chapelhow, C. and Crouch, C. (2007) 'Applying numeracy skills in clinical practice: fluid balance'. *Nursing Standard*, 21(27): 49–56
This article applies SI units and numeracy skills to the measurement and

calculation of fluid intake and output using clinical scenarios. Informative, as well as providing some practice questions.

Myers, H. (2003) 'Hospital fall risk assessment tools: A critique of the literature'. *International Journal of Nursing Practice*, 9(4): 223–35
A thorough critique of the literature relating to risk assessment tools used to predict falls in hospital. The complexities of designing risk assessment tools are revealed. Challenges, like methodological problems and the lack of adequate testing, that face nurses when trying to implement evidence-informed practice are explored.

Pancorbo-Hidalgo, P.L., Garcia-Fernandez, F.P., Lopez-Medina, I.M. and Alvarez-Nieto, C. (2006) 'Risk assessment scales for pressure ulcer prevention: a systematic review'. *Journal of Advanced Nursing*, 54(1): 94–110
This is a thorough analysis of research studies undertaken to establish the effectiveness of pressure ulcer risk assessment calculators. The article examines the problems of accuracy and 'cut-off scores'.

www.bapen.org.uk/must_tool.html
This is the MUST tool website. It provides details of the MUST tool, BMI and weight loss charts, as well as a considerable amount of additional information relating to nutritional support.

Chapter 6

An Introduction to Measurement and Basic Statistics

> **INTRODUCTION**
>
> Nurses and other health care professionals need to understand simple statistics to help them interpret and evaluate research reports. This chapter introduces the numerical basis of simple statistics and measurement. The application, strengths and weaknesses of measures of central tendency and dispersion are considered as calculations that are used to describe data. Probability is introduced as one of the fundamental properties of **inferential statistics** and the meaning of levels of significance is explained.

NUMBERS, NURSES AND STATISTICS

There are concerns about nurses' numeracy skills (Jukes and Gilchrist, 2006; Department of Health, 2004b). However, the evidence for these concerns is usually obtained through theoretical tests (Kapborg, 1994; Bliss-Holtz, 1994; Blais and Bath, 1992). The reality of clinical practice is not about sitting a numeracy examination, but using numeracy skills accurately in clinical practice to ensure patient safety. Numeracy skills need to be viewed as an integral part of clinical practice. The intention of previous chapters has been to show how an understanding of the essential components of numeracy, like the SI system of measurement, performing drug and nutritional calculations contributes to everyday health care.

Professional practice should be informed and guided by the best available evidence and numeracy skills are needed as part of this process. Whether you are a pre-registration student nurse, returning to health care following a career break or simply 'brushing up' on your numeracy skills, there is an expectation that modern practice is based, wherever possible, on one of the most significant sources of evidence – research. This involves reading research reports. The phrase 'reading research' sounds straightforward and rather painless. However, there is a great deal more to this than the reading skills that most of us will have acquired over the years spent at school. Reading research depends on a knowledge base and several fundamental skills that modern health care staff need to have in their 'professional toolkit'. These include:

- the ability to access and search databases;
- an understanding of the research process and methodologies;
- an ability to read critically;
- an understanding of the way that findings may be arrived at and presented – statistics.

Numeracy skills are one of several fundamental skills that allow nurses to read research reports and to make decisions about the use of research findings in practice.

WHAT ARE STATISTICS?

In Chapter One, nurses were considered as being 'typical of the population as a whole in that many are not good at numerical calculations' (Hutton, 2000, p. 894). From my experience of teaching numeracy and drug calculations to nurses and other health care professionals, they tend to fall into one of two camps – those who are aware that they have some skills and those who, usually wrongly, believe they are hopeless cases. Statistics can cause similar feelings. Nurses and other health care professionals don't have the option of choosing to develop an understanding of statistics or not; modern health care demands that they acquire this skill, usually in educational programmes that lead to registration. Pre-registration courses or post-registration modules will also introduce the reading and critiquing skills necessary to help you to become research-aware.

Statistics and measurement

The word 'statistics' has two meanings. It can refer to **quantitative** information or **data**, or it can mean the specific tests that can be used to examine quantitative data. Health care professionals gather quantitative data from patients daily and sometimes more frequently. Physiological measurements like blood pressure, blood glucose levels, temperature, body weight, fluid intake and output are all quantitative data relating to individual patients, although we may not think about these 'routine measurements' in such grand terms. Interestingly, we may shudder at the mention of the word statistics, yet we use them within everyday practice without a second thought. In clinical practice statistics have a value in that they allow us to describe some characteristics of a patient and communicate these to others. Similarly, statistics used in research have the same value in that they allow the researcher to summarise some characteristics of a **sample** or **variable**, and allow this to be communicated in a standard form.

Measurements are a feature of clinical practice that we accept almost without question. Patients might be asked to rate their satisfaction with the health services and care they have received. When you have attended a study day an evaluation or measurement of your satisfaction with the day is routine. We try to measure how much pain a patient is suffering or measure the risk of certain events like sustaining a fall or developing a pressure ulcer. Variables (like age, weight, gender and height) measured in the clinical environment can be divided into two broad categories, continuous and discrete.

Continuous variables

Continuous means that the measurement of the variable can fall at any point on a continuous scale. Scales that can be thought of as continuous have already been mentioned in earlier chapters. Weight measured in kilograms and grams and pH as a measurement of hydrogen ion concentration are both examples of continuous scales. Many other variables are measured on continuous scales in clinical practice including temperature, blood glucose levels and blood pressure. All of these scales have set numerical points with 'in between' values. When measuring a patient's weight, this could be 72.5 kg, halfway between 72 kg and 73 kg.

Discrete variables

Variables classified as discrete can only be expressed as separate categories. If you were to record information about a patient's blood group, the available categories would include:

- A rhesus positive;
- A rhesus negative;
- B rhesus positive;
- B rhesus negative;
- O rhesus positive;
- O rhesus negative.

Patients can only fit into one category and there are no 'in between' values. Other examples of variables that can be classed as discrete are nationality and gender. Sometimes you may see discrete data referred to as 'discontinuous data'.

Levels of measurement

The nature of variables relates to how they can be measured. There are four levels of measurement: **nominal**, **ordinal**, **interval** and **ratio**. These are related to statistics as well as scales used in clinical practice. It is important to appreciate that each level of measurement has rules about its use.

Nominal measurement

Nominal measurement can barely be thought of as measuring as it is simply assigning a variable to a category. This process is really 'naming'. For example, if you wanted to find out what type of blood group a patient was, you could ask them if they knew or you could send a sample of blood to the laboratory for grouping. This could then be documented. Sometimes nominal categories have numbers assigned to them as below:

1. A rhesus positive;
2. A rhesus negative;
3. B rhesus positive;
4. B rhesus negative;
5. O rhesus positive;
6. O rhesus negative.

The numbers have no numerical value; they are only used to label the categories.

Example 1
The enrolment form at a weight reduction clinic asks participants to identify their gender. It asks:
Are you:
1. Male
or
2. Female

If six males and 18 females attended the clinic, the only calculation possible is a percentage distribution. This involves calculating the number of men and women who attended as a percentage of the total number of attendees.

To calculate the percentage of men = $\dfrac{\text{Number of men}}{\text{Total attending the clinic}} \times 100$

$= \dfrac{6 \times 100}{24} = 25$

So 25% of the clinic attendees were male.

To calculate the percentage of women = $\dfrac{\text{Number of women}}{\text{Total attending the clinic}} \times 100$

$= \dfrac{18}{24} \times 100 = 75$

So 75% of the clinic attendees were female.

Ordinal measurement

Ordinal measurement is one step further up the hierarchy than nominal. At this level of measurement, the category is named and there is some meaningful order or ranking. For example, a dependency scale might contain the following categories:

1. Immobile;
2. Can mobilise with carers and walking aids;
3. Mobile with walking aids;
4. Mobilises independently.

In this example there is a progression along the scale from immobile to independence, but it is not possible to accurately express the difference between each measurement on the scale. Ordinal scales are commonly used in health care; clinical risk assessment scales like pressure ulcer assessment calculators frequently incorporate an ordinal scale. Evaluation tools used to measure patient satisfaction with care, or the measurement of student satisfaction with educational experiences, both clinical and theoretical, can also involve ordinal scales. In these examples there is often an arbitrary point, for example 80%, which is regarded as being acceptable. Scores below this level would indicate dissatisfaction. Using ordinal scales in this manner can be criticised as they are intended to measure rank order. In Chapter Five, similar criticisms were made about pressure ulcer risk calculators having absolute 'cut-off points' above which patients would develop pressure ulcers.

Interval measurement

Interval measurement, in addition to progression in the order of measurement, identifies with precision the difference between each unit on the scale. On interval scales, the zero point is not absolute and can't be taken to mean that there is an absence of the variable. If days are used as an example, the difference between 30 March and 31 March is exactly the same as that between 7 February and 8 February. There is no zero point. Temperature is another example of an interval scale. When measuring temperature in degrees Celsius, the zero point on the scale is the point at which water freezes, but temperature doesn't cease to exist at this point, hence the phrase 'sub-zero temperatures'. Because the difference between each point on an interval scale is exact, most mathematical calculations can be performed on interval level data, unlike nominal and ordinal data. But, as the zero point is not absolute, it cannot be said that 16 degrees Celsius is twice as hot as 8 degrees Celsius.

Ratio measurement

Ratio measurement is at the top of the hierarchy of measurement. This level of measurement incorporates the properties of nominal, ordinal and interval scales, but also has an absolute zero. This allows all mathematical procedures to be performed as well as knowing that, for example, a weight of 12 kg is four times that of 3 kg. Scales that measure weight and height are examples of ratio scales. Often ratio and interval scales are grouped together as there is little difference between the two.

RESEARCH AND STATISTICS

Research methods can be classified into two general approaches, **qualitative methods** and **quantitative methods**. Qualitative methods seek to find understanding of individuals or events and produce data in text form, rather than numbers. Quantitative methods aim to measure variables or to identify relationships between them, by collecting and analysing data and identifying and describing numerical relationships and patterns. A study designed to answer the question 'how many hours do patients spend asleep in hospital at night?' would produce quantitative data relating to the amount of time spent sleeping. A study asking 'what influence does pain have on the amount of time spent asleep by hospital patients?' would produce quantitative data that may indicate a relationship between pain and sleep.

In quantitative studies data is analysed numerically so, when reading quantitative research, you need to ask 'is it clear how the data was analysed?' and 'if any statistical tests were used, what is the purpose of these, and what are they trying to explain?'. In keeping with many subjects, research and statistics have their own vocabulary and specialist terminology that needs to be learned. This involves reading research reports, making notes about research methods or statistics that you are unclear about, and then referring to the glossary found in any good research textbook. Health care professionals are regularly faced with

Measures of dispersion

As well as knowing the average values in a data set, it is also necessary to understand how the data is spread. This is also called variance. Measures of dispersion are calculations that help interpret research findings, particularly when trying to compare two or more sets of data. Measures of dispersion include the range, interquartile range and standard deviation.

Range

On data that has been obtained at ordinal level, the range is calculated as the 'least to the greatest score'. In the student nurse drug calculation test the range would be expressed as 3–19. When the data has been measured at interval or ratio level, the range is calculated as 'the difference between the greatest and the least score'. Using the same drug test results as an example, the range would be calculated as: $19 - 3 = 16$.

Interquartile range

When calculating the range, only the two extreme values are used. One way of overcoming this is to calculate the interquartile range, which considers values a quarter and three-quarters of the way up the data set. This provides a better description of the spread or variance of the data as it ignores the lowest and highest values, and is based around the median. If you recall, the median was the mid-point in a range of data with 50% of the scores falling below it and 50% above. The lower quartile, also known as the first quartile, is calculated as the mid-point between the lowest score and the median, with 25% of the scores lying below this point. The upper quartile, also called the third quartile, is the mid-point between the median and the highest score, and 75% of scores will fall below this point. The interquartile range is from the first quartile to the third quartile and because it is based on middle scores, rather than extremes, it is considered to be more stable.

Standard deviation

The standard deviation is a calculation that considers the extent to which, on average, every value in a data set deviates from the mean. It can be calculated using interval or ratio level data. The benefit of this as a measure of dispersion is that a standard deviation considers all of the values, whereas calculating the range considers only two values from a data set that are at the extremes and these could be atypical. If the standard deviation is small then this indicates that the values are relatively close to the mean. If the standard deviation is large, this suggests that the values are more widely spread. Standard deviation is usually abbreviated to 's', and modern scientific calculators mean that it is rarely necessary to perform the calculation longhand.

Correlation

Correlation describes the relationship between two variables or two sets of results, and can be calculated with data obtained on ordinal, interval or ratio scales. Using the previous example of the first-year student nurse drug calculation test results, a researcher might be interested to see if there is a relationship between previous mathematics qualifications such as GCSE at grade C or above, and the scores in the drug test. If the results indicated that those student nurses who achieved the highest grades at GCSE also achieved the highest results in the drug calculation test, this would indicate a perfect correlation and is expressed as '1'. If there were no correlation, this would be expressed as '0'. If it were found that those who achieved the highest grades at GCSE scored lowest on the test, this would indicate a negative correlation, which is expressed as '-1'. When reading a research report that refers to correlations, do remember that just because there is a relationship between two sets of data, it does not follow that one has caused the other. This could be purely coincidental or due to other variables. Descriptive statistics such as correlations do not seek to identify a cause and effect relationship, but merely to establish that a relationship exists. **Inferential statistics** examine the nature of relationships between variables.

Normal distribution

An awareness of normal distribution is useful as it helps to understand measures of central tendency, standard deviation and some aspects of inferential statistics. For example, if sufficient blood glucose measurements were taken from a large group of people and then plotted on a graph, the result would take the shape of a bell-shaped curve or normal distribution curve. Figure 1 below shows that, in a normal population, most of the results fall in the middle area. In fact, 68% of all measurements are within one standard deviation of the mean, 34% above and 34% below. Overall, approximately 95% of all of the measurements will be within two standard deviations of the mean, with only a small number (about 4%) at the extremes. In a normal distribution the mean, median and mode are the same. Other measurements like height, intelligence, weight and blood pressure would follow the same pattern as blood glucose.

6. A patient takes three 30 mcg tablets daily. She plans to go on holiday and will take enough tablets for 14 days. Expressed in mg, how much of the drug will she take with her?
Answer = 1.26 mg

7. The local health centre is open Monday to Friday each week. The domestic mops the corridor floor and waiting area twice each day using 0.275 L of cleaning fluid each time. The cleaning fluid is supplied in containers that hold 4 500 ml.
Expressed in ml and L, how much cleaning fluid will be left in the container at the end of the week?
Answer = The domestic uses 550 ml per day for five days of the week.
550 × 5 = 2 750 ml.
4 500 ml – 2 750 = 1 750 ml or 1.75 L

8. A liquid medicine contains 20 mg in 5 ml
a. How many mg are in 25 ml?
Answer = 5 × 20 = 100 mg

b. How many mg are in 2.5 ml?
Answer = 0.5 × 20 = 10 mg

c. How many mg are in 7.5 ml?
Answer = 1.5 × 20 = 30 mg

Chapter Four

Calculating tablets:
1. A patient is prescribed 5 mg of bendroflumethiazide. How many 2.5 mg tablets should be given?
Answer: 2 tablets, because 2 × 2.5 mg = 5 mg

2. A patient is prescribed 7.5 mg of soluble prednisolone orally. How many 5 mg tablets should be given?
Answer: 1.5 tablets, because 1.5 × 5 mg = 7.5 mg

3. A patient is prescribed 120 mg of furosemide. How many 40 mg tablets should be given?
Answer: 3 tablets, because 3 × 40 mg = 120 mg

4. A patient is prescribed 250 micrograms of digoxin. How many 125 microgram tablets should be given?
Answer: 2 tablets, because 2 × 125 micrograms = 250 micrograms

5. A patient is prescribed 40 mg of gliclazide. How many 80 mg tablets should be given?

Answer 0.5 of a tablet, because 0.5×80 mg = 40 mg

Calculating liquid medicines

1. An adult is prescribed 300 mg of sodium valproate oral solution. The bottle label states there are 200 mg in 5 ml. What volume of sodium valproate needs to be administered?

Using the WIG equation:

Want = 300 mg

In = 5 ml

Got = 200 mg

$$\frac{300 \times 5}{200} = \frac{1\,500}{200} = 7.5 \text{ ml}$$

2. A child is prescribed 12 mg of furosemide oral solution. The bottle label states there are 8 mg per ml. What volume of sodium furosemide needs to be administered?

Using the WIG equation:

Want = 12 mg

In = 1 ml

Got = 8 mg

$$\frac{12 \times 1}{8} = 1.5 \text{ ml}$$

3. A child is prescribed 62.5 mg of phenoxymethylpenicillin (Penicillin V) oral solution. The bottle label states there are 125 mg in 5 ml. What volume of phenoxymethylpenicillin needs to be administered?

Using the WIG equation:

Want = 62.5 mg

In = 5 ml

Got = 125 mg

$$\frac{62.5 \times 5}{125} = \frac{312.5}{125} = 2.5 \text{ ml}$$

4. A patient is prescribed 210 mg of ferrous fumarate syrup. The bottle label states there are 140 mg in 5 ml. What volume of ferrous fumarate needs to be administered?

Using the WIG equation:

Want = 210 mg

In = 5 ml

Got = 140 mg

$$\frac{210 \times 5}{140} = \frac{1\,050}{140} = 7.5 \text{ ml}$$

5. A patient is prescribed 750 ml of intravenous Ringer's solution to run over 3 hours.
    What volume of fluid should run hourly?
    Using the equation:
    $$\frac{\text{Volume to be infused (ml)}}{\text{Duration of infusion (hours)}} = \text{ml per hour}$$

    $750 \div 3 = 250$ ml / hour

Intravenous infusion drop rates

1. A patient is prescribed 1 000 ml of intravenous Sodium Chloride 0.9% to run over 6 hours. Using a standard intravenous infusion set, how many drops per minute are needed to infuse the fluid over the prescribed time?
    Using the equation:
    $$\frac{\text{Volume prescribed (ml)}}{\text{Hours of infusion}} \times \frac{\text{Drops per ml of administration set}}{\text{60 minutes}}$$

    $\dfrac{1\,000}{6} \times \dfrac{20}{60} = 166.6$ (recurring) $\times 0.33$ (recurring) $= 55$ drops per min

2. A patient is prescribed 500 ml of intravenous Dextrose 5% to run over 4 hours. Using a standard intravenous infusion set, how many drops per minute are needed to infuse the fluid over the prescribed time?
    Using the equation:
    $$\frac{\text{Volume prescribed (ml)}}{\text{Hours of infusion}} \times \frac{\text{Drops per ml of administration set}}{\text{60 minutes}}$$

    $\dfrac{500}{4} \times \dfrac{20}{60} = 125 \times 0.33$ (recurring) $= 41$ drops per minute

3. A patient is prescribed 1 000 ml of intravenous Ringer's solution to run over 8 hours. Using a standard intravenous infusion set, how many drops per minute are needed to infuse the fluid over the prescribed time?
    Using the equation:
    $$\frac{\text{Volume prescribed (ml)}}{\text{Hours of infusion}} \times \frac{\text{Drops per ml of administration set}}{\text{60 minutes}}$$

    $\dfrac{1\,000}{8} \times \dfrac{20}{60} = 125 \times 0.33$ (recurring) $= 41$ drops per minute

4. A patient is prescribed 500 ml of intravenous Sodium Chloride 0.9% to run over 6 hours.
    Using a standard intravenous infusion set, how many drops per minute are needed to infuse the fluid over the prescribed time?
    Using the equation:

    $$\frac{\text{Volume prescribed (ml)}}{\text{Hours of infusion}} \times \frac{\text{Drops per ml of administration set}}{\text{60 minutes}}$$

    $$\frac{500}{6} \times \frac{20}{60} = 83.3 \text{ (recurring)} \times 0.33 \text{ (recurring)} = 27 \text{ drops per minute}$$

5. A patient is prescribed 750 ml of intravenous Ringer's solution to run over 3 hours.
    Using a standard intravenous infusion set, how many drops per minute are needed to infuse the fluid over the prescribed time?
    Using the equation:

    $$\frac{\text{Volume prescribed (ml)}}{\text{Hours of infusion}} \times \frac{\text{Drops per ml of administration set}}{\text{60 minutes}}$$

    $$\frac{750}{3} \times \frac{20}{60} = 250 \times 0.33 \text{ (recurring)} = 83 \text{ drops per minute}$$

Dose per kg of body weight calculations:
1. A patient is prescribed 5 mcg of digoxin per kilogram of body weight. If the patient weighs 76 kg what amount of digoxin needs to be given? Digoxin is available in ampoules containing 500 mcg in 2 ml. What is the volume of digoxin that needs to be given?
    Using the equation:
    Dose to be administered = Patient's weight × Dose per kg
    $76 \times 5 = 380$ mcg
    To determine the amount needing to be administered, the WIG equation is used:

    $$\frac{380 \times 2}{500} = \frac{760}{500} = 1.52 \text{ ml}$$

2. A patient is prescribed an injection of midazolam intramuscularly at 80 mcg per kilogram of body weight.
    If the patient weighs 75 kg what amount of midazolam needs to be given?
    Midazolam is available in ampoules containing 10 mg in 2 ml (5 mg per ml). What is the volume of midazolam that needs to be given?
    Using the equation:
    Dose to be administered = Patient's weight × Dose per kg
    $75 \times 80 = 6\ 000$ mcg or 6 mg
    To determine the amount needing to be administered, the WIG

equation is used:

$$\frac{6 \times 2}{10} = \frac{12}{10} = 1.2 \text{ ml}$$

3. A patient is prescribed enoxaparin at 1.5 mg (150 units) per kilogram of body weight.

   If the patient weighs 70 kg what amount of enoxaparin needs to be given?

   Enoxaparin is available as 120 mg (12 000 units) in 0.8 ml. What volume of enoxaparin needs to be given?

   Using the equation:

   Dose to be administered = Patient's weight × Dose per kg

   $70 \times 150 = 10\ 500$ units

   To determine the amount needing to be administered, the WIG equation is used:

   $$\frac{10\ 500 \times 0.8}{12\ 000} = \frac{8\ 400}{12\ 000} = 0.7 \text{ ml}$$

4. A nine-month-old baby weighs 8.5 kg and is prescribed morphine at 200 mcg per kilogram of body weight. What amount of morphine needs to be administered?

   Morphine is available as 10 mg in 1 ml. What volume needs to be given?

   Using the equation:

   Dose to be administered = Patient's weight x Dose per kg

   $8.5 \times 200 = 1\ 700$ mcg or 1.7 mg

   To determine the amount needing to be administered, the WIG equation is used:

   $$\frac{1.7 \times 1}{10} = 0.17 \text{ ml}$$

5. A patient is prescribed 5 mg of gentamicin per kilogram of body weight.

   If the patient weighs 84 kg what is the total daily amount of gentamicin to be given?

   If there are three equal doses per day, how many milligrams of gentamicin are given at each dose?

   Gentamicin is stocked in vials of 80 mg in 2 ml. What is the volume of gentamicin to be given at each dose?

   Using the equation:

   Dose to be administered = Patient's weight × Dose per kg

   $84 \times 5 = 420$ mg (total daily amount)

   $420 \div 3 = 140$ mg (each dose)

   To determine the amount needing to be administered, the WIG equation is used:

$$140 \times 2 = \frac{280}{80} = 3.5 \text{ ml}$$

Chapter Five

Fluid balance chart calculations
1. The total oral intake = 1 950 ml
2. The total intravenous intake = 400 ml
3. The total fluid intake = 2 350 ml
4. The total urine output = 2 430 ml
5. The total fluid output = 2 480 ml
6. The fluid balance for this 24 hour period = input − output = -130 ml (negative)

BMI calculations
1. A male patient is 1.84 m tall and weighs 96 kg. What is his BMI?
$$\frac{96}{1.84 \times 1.84} = \frac{96}{3.3856} = 28.35 = \text{BMI } 28$$

2. A female patient is 1.66 m tall and weighs 58 kg. What is her BMI?
$$\frac{58}{1.66 \times 1.66} = \frac{58}{2.7556} = 21.04 = \text{BMI } 21$$

3. A male patient is 1.78 m tall and weighs 77 kg. What is his BMI?
$$\frac{77}{1.78 \times 1.78} = \frac{77}{3.1684} = 24.3 = \text{BMI } 24$$

4. A female patient is 1.56 m tall and weighs 47 kg. What is her BMI?
$$\frac{47}{1.56 \times 1.56} = \frac{47}{2.4336} = 19.31 = \text{BMI } 19$$

5. A female patient is 1.72 m tall and weighs 89 kg. What is her BMI?
$$\frac{89}{1.72 \times 1.72} = \frac{89}{2.9584} = 30.08 = \text{BMI } 30$$

MUST score risk calculations
1. A male patient is 1.78 m tall and weighs 65 kg. He is able to eat and drink normally, but has unintentionally lost 5 kg over the last four months. Using the MUST tool, calculate his level of risk.
   BMI = 21 = score 0
   Weight loss score = 1
   Total = 1 = Medium risk

2. A female patient is 1.68 m tall and weighs 54 kg. She is able to eat and drink normally, but over the last three months has unintentionally lost 6 kg.
   Using the MUST tool, calculate her level of risk.
   BMI = 19 = score 1
   Weight loss score = 2
   Total = 3 = High risk

3. A male patient is 1.76 m tall and weighs 60 kg. He has a raised body temperature and abdominal pain, and has eaten very little over the past week. During the last four months, he has noticed that his weight has decreased from 62 kg, without dieting. Using the MUST tool, calculate his level of risk.
   BMI = 19 = score 1
   Weight loss score (less than 5%) = score 0
   Unable to eat over the last week = score 2
   Total = 3 = High risk

4. A female patient is 1.6 m tall and weighs 80 kg. She is admitted with a history of developing a chest infection after a bout of influenza approximately six weeks ago. It is thought that she has developed pneumonia. Her appetite has decreased over the last two weeks and she has not eaten anything substantial for the last four days.
   Using the MUST tool, calculate her level of risk.
   BMI = 31 (obese) = score 0
   No weight loss
   Acutely ill / unable to eat = score 2
   Total = 2 = High risk.

Ideal body weight calculations
Calculate the ideal body weight for the following:
1. A female who is 1.6 m (5 feet 3 inches) tall.
   The first 1.52 m (5 ft) of height = 45.5 kg [100 lb] + (3 × 2.3 kg) [3 × 5 lb] = 52.4 kg [8 stone 3 lb]
2. A male who is 1.78 m (5 feet 10 inches) tall.
   The first 1.52 m, (5 ft) of height = 48 kg [106 lb] + (10 × 2.5 kg) [10 × 6 lb] = 73 kg [11 stone 12 lb]
3. A female who is 1.68 m (5 feet 6 inches) tall.
   The first 1.52 m (5 ft) of height = 45.5 kg [100 lb] + (6 × 2.3 kg) [6 × 5 lb] = 59.3 kg [9 stone 4 lb]
4. A male who is 1.7 m (5 feet 7 inches) tall.
   The first 1.52 m (5 ft) of height = 48 kg [106 lb] + (7 × 2.5 kg) [7 × 6 lb] = 65.5 kg [10 stone 8 lb]

Glossary

Acid A substance that releases hydrogen ions.

Alkaline A substance that releases ions that can combine with hydrogen ions.

Antibiotic A drug that has a direct toxic effect on bacteria.

Arithmetical Relating to the use of numbers in counting and calculation.

Cannula A narrow bore, flexible plastic tube that is inserted through the skin and into a vein to allow the administration of intravenous fluids or medication.

Capsules Surrounded by a hard coat, capsules are oval shaped and may contain powdered or liquid medicines which taste unpleasant, or could irritate the mouth and upper part of the gastrointestinal tract.

Chemotherapy The use of cytotoxic drugs to destroy malignant (cancer) cells. Lower doses of some cytotoxic drugs are used in the treatment of some non-cancerous conditions such as psoriasis and rheumatoid arthritis.

Clinical outcome A component of clinically based learning that a student is required to achieve in order to register. Several related outcomes are grouped together to form the proficiencies for entry to the register.

Clinical risk assessment calculators A variety of tools designed to measure the risk that a patient has of developing a condition such as pressure ulcers, sustaining a fall or needing high dependency care.

Cytotoxic agent A drug designed to destroy malignant cells and used as chemotherapy. Can also damage all rapidly dividing cells, malignant or non-malignant.

Data Data are pieces of information that can be obtained by enquiry, as in patient assessment, or during the course of a research study.

Decimals Decimals are the units within the decimal system; a number system based on units of 10.

Narrow therapeutic range The therapeutic range of a drug is where most users will receive the clinical effect, with few adverse effects. This is between the lower concentrations of the drug in the blood stream where there will be minimal drug effect, and the upper concentrations where there is an increasing probability of adverse effects. Minor fluctuations in blood levels of drugs with a narrow therapeutic range caused by variations to the administration frequency or absorption of the drug, could result in the drug failing to achieve a therapeutic effect, or lead to adverse effects.

Nebuliser solution A mixture of a drug and a solution, for example salbutamol and 0.9% Sodium Chloride, which is converted into a fine spray and inhaled via a face mask or mouthpiece.

Nominal The most basic level of measurement or scale, where variables are assigned to a named category.

Non-parametric A group of inferential statistical tests that are used to examine the relationships between variables when data may not meet the assumptions required for parametric tests.

Numeracy Skills that relate to a good basic knowledge of arithmetic; being numerate.

Numerator The top number in a fraction.

Oedema Excess interstitial fluid (surrounding the cells) caused by an increased water and sodium content.

Oral medicines A name for medicines that are ingested via the mouth including tablets, capsules and liquids. Some drugs are taken via sublingual or buccal routes, and although these are part of the oral cavity, these medicines are not swallowed.

Ordinal A scale or measurement where there is naming and ranking, but the difference between each point of measurement is not exact.

Parametric A group of inferential statistical tests that have rigorous assumptions about the distribution of variables in a population, and require interval or ratio level measurement.

pascal SI unit of pressure also used in clinical practice.

Patch A self-adhesive patch containing drugs that are absorbable through the skin. Usually applied to hairless areas of the body such as the abdomen or chest.

Percentage A common way of expressing values 'for each hundred'. Useful in making comparisons.

pH scale A scale that measures how acid or alkaline a solution is.

Population The total number of individuals from which data could be collected.

Power A way of expressing very large or small numbers, which reduces the number of zeros that need to be written.

Proper fraction A fraction where the numerator is smaller than the denominator, e.g. ½.

Psoriasis A chronic skin disease characterised by the build-up of a white, waxy silver scale on the skin.

Qualitative Qualitative data are non-numerical.

Qualitative methods A research approach that investigates feelings, beliefs or attitudes and seeks to understand reality.

Quantitative Information or data in numerical form.

Quantitative methods A research approach that measures variables and/or the relationships between them.

Ratio A value that indicates a relationship or comparison between two items.

Ratio (statistical) A category of measurement or scale where there is progression in the order of measurement, the difference between each point on the scale is exact and there is a true zero point.

Rheumatoid arthritis A systemic disease of connective tissue causing inflammatory changes and damage to synovial joints and tendon sheaths.

Sample A subset of the population used within a research study.

Variable A characteristic of an object or person that varies, for example age, blood pressure, eye colour or weight.

Vincristine A potent cytotoxic drug used in the treatment of some types of leukaemia, lymphomas and lung and breast cancer.

Volumetric pump An electronic pump that dispenses a controlled and continuous flow of intravenous fluid.

References

Allibone, L. and Nation, N. (2006) 'A guide to regulation of blood gases: part 2'. *Nursing Times*, 102(46): 48–50

Audit Commission (2001) *Spoonful of sugar – medicines management in NHS hospitals*. London: Audit Commission

Bell, J. (2007), 'Nutritional screening during hospital admission: part 2'. *Nursing Times*, 103(38): 30–31

Blais, K. and Bath, J.B. (1992) 'Drug calculation errors of baccalaureate nursing students'. *Nurse Educator*, 17(1): 12–15

Bliss-Holtz, J. (1994) 'Discriminating types of medication calculation errors in nursing practice'. *Nursing Research*, 43(6): 373–5

Bowling, T. (2004), *Nutritional Support for Adults and Children*. Oxford: Radcliffe Medical Press

Bryant, H. (2007) 'Dehydration in older people: assessment and management'. *Emergency Nurse*, 5(4): 22–6

Cartwright, M. (1996) 'Numeracy needs of the beginning Registered Nurse'. *Nurse Education Today*, 16: 137–43

Castledine, G. (2006) 'Nurse whose attitude towards drug administration put patients at risk'. *British Journal of Nursing*, 15(1): 29

Cooper, M. (1995) 'Can a zero defects philosophy be applied to drug errors?' *Journal of Advanced Nursing*, 21: 487–91

Department of Health (2000) *An organization with a memory*. London: HMSO

Department of Health (2004a) *Building a Safer NHS for patients: Improving Medication Safety*. London: HMSO

Department of Health (2004b) *National Service Framework for Children, Young People and Maternity Services Standard 10 Medicines for Children and Young People*. London: HMSO

Eaton, N. (1997) 'Parametric data analysis'. *Nurse Researcher*, 4(4): 17–27

Elia, M. (2003), *Screening for Malnutrition: A Multidisciplinary Responsibility. Development and use of the Malnutrition Universal Screening Tool (MUST) for adults*. Maidenhead: British Association for Parenteral and Enteral Nutrition

Fulbrook, P., Bongers, A. and Albarran, J. (2007) 'A European survey of enteral nutrition practices and procedures in adult intensive care units'. *Journal of Clinical Nursing*, 16(11): 2132–41

Goldhill, D., Singh, S., Tarling, M., Worthington, L., Mulcahy, A., White, S. and Sumner, A. (1999) 'The patient at risk team: identifying and managing seriously ill ward patients'. *Anaesthesia*, 54: 853–60

Grandell-Niemi, H., Hupli, M., Puukka, P. and Leino-Kilpi, H. (2006) 'Finnish nurses' and nursing students' mathematical skills'. *Nurse Education Today*, 26(2): 151–61

Haigh, S. (2002) 'How to calculate drug dosage accurately: advice for nurses'. *Professional Nurse*, 18(1): 54–7

Hall, C. (2006) 'A third of new nurses fail simple English and maths test.' *Daily Telegraph*, Saturday 5 August, p.8

Hallett, C. (1997) 'The use of descriptive statistics in nursing research'. *Nurse Researcher*, 4(4): 4–16

Higgins, D. (2005) 'Drug calculations'. *Nursing Times*, 101(46): 24–5

Holman, C., Roberts, S. and Nicol, M. (2005) 'Promoting adequate hydration in older people'. *Nursing Older People*, 17(4): 31–2

Hutton, B.M. (1998) 'Do school qualifications predict competence in nursing calculations?' *Nurse Education Today*, 18: 25–31

Hutton, B.M. (2000) 'Numeracy must become a priority for nurses'. *British Journal of Nursing*, 9(14): 894

Johnstone, C., Farley, A. and Hendry, C. (2006) 'Nurses' role in nutritional assessment and screening' (part one). *Nursing Times*, 102(49) 28–9

Jukes, L. and Gilchrist, M. (2006) 'Concerns about numeracy skills of nursing students'. *Nurse Education in Practice*, 6(4): 192–98

Kapborg, I.D. (1994) 'Calculation and administration of drug dosage by Swedish nurses, student nurses and physicians.' *International Journal for Quality in Health Care*, 6(4): 389–95

Lecko, C. (2006) 'We can no longer blame the quality of hospital food for malnutrition in hospitals'. *Nursing Times*, 102(9): 12

Lerwill, C.J. (1999) 'Ability and attitudes to mathematics of post-registration health-care professional'. *Nurse Education Today*, 19: 319–22

Lindsay, B. (2007) *Understanding Research and Evidence-based Practice*. Exeter: Reflect Press Ltd

Malnutrition Advisory Group (2003a) 'A consistent and reliable tool for malnutrition screening'. *Nursing Times*, 99(46): 26–7

Malnutrition Advisory Group (2003b) 'Malnutrition universal screening tool' **www. bapen.org.uk/must_tool.html** (accessed 3 January 2008)

Metheny, N.A., Dettenmeter, P., Hampton, K., Wiersma, L. and Williams, P. (1990) 'Detection of inadvertent respiratory placement of small bore feeding tubes. A report of 10 cases'. *Heart and Lung*, 19: 631–8

Miller, J.A. (1992) 'Can nurses do their sums?' *Nursing Times*, 88(32): 40–41

McAtear, C.A. (2006) 'Malnutrition in hospitals. What can you and I do?' *British Journal of Nursing*, 15(20): 1090

McWhirter, J.P. and Pennington, C.R. (1994) 'Incidence and recognition of malnutrition in hospital'. *British Medical Journal*, 308: 945–8

Montague, S.E., Watson, R. and Herbert, R.A. (2005), *Physiology for Nursing Practice* (3rd edition). Edinburgh: Elsevier

National Institute for Clinical Excellence (2003) *The use of pressure relieving devices (beds, mattresses, and overlays) for the prevention of pressure ulcers in primary and secondary care.* London: NICE

National Patient Safety Agency (2005) Alert No. 5 February **www.npsa.nhs.uk**

National Patient Safety Agency (2007a) Nasogastric Tube Incidents: Summary Update **www.npsa.nhs.uk**

National Patient Safety Agency (2007b) New toolkit encourages good hydration for hospital patients **www.npsa.nhs.uk**

Nightingale, F. (1859) (reprinted 1970) *Notes on Nursing: What It Is and What It Is Not.* Glasgow: Blackie

Norton, D., Mclaren, R. and Exton-Smith, A.N. (1975) *An investigation of geriatric nursing problems in hospital.* Edinburgh: Churchill Livingstone

Nursing and Midwifery Council (2004) Standards of proficiency for pre-registration midwifery education **www.nmc-uk.org**

Nursing and Midwifery Council (2007a) Essential Skills Clusters (circular 07/2007, annexes 1, 2 and 3) available at: **www.nmc-uk.org** (accessed 3 January 2008)

Nursing and Midwifery Council (2007b) *Standards for medicines management* available at: **www.nmc-uk.org** (accessed 14 February 2008)

Nutrition Now (2007) 'Drink to good health'. *Nursing Standard*, 22(2): 17-21

Office for National Statistics (ONS) (2006) *Social Trends 36*. Basingstoke: Palgrave Macmillan.

Palmer, R. (2004) 'Using an early warning system in a medical assessment unit'. *Nursing Times*, 100:48 34-35

Pancorbo-Hidalgo, P.L., Garcia-Fernandez, F.P., Lopez-Medina, I.M. and Alvarez-Nieto, C. (2006) 'Risk assessment scales for pressure ulcer prevention: a systematic review'. *Journal of Advanced Nursing*, 54(1): 94–110

Pentin, J. and Smith, J. (2006) 'Drug calculations: are they safer with or without a calculator?' *British Journal of Nursing*, 15(14): 778–81

Sandwell, M. and Carson, P. (2005) 'Developing numeracy in child branch students'. *Paediatric Nursing*, 17(9) 24–6

Thompson, D. (2005) 'An evaluation of the Waterlow Pressure ulcer risk assessment tool'. *British Journal of Nursing*, 14 (18): 455–9

Trim, J. (2004) 'Clinical skills: a practical guide to working out drug calculations'. *British Journal of Nursing*, 13(10): 602–6

Watson, H. (1997) 'Nonparametric data analysis'. *Nurse Researcher*, 4(4): 28–40

Watson, R., Atkinson, I. and Egerton, P. (2006) *Successful Statistics for Healthcare*. Basingstoke: Palgrave Macmillan

Weeks, K., Lyne, P. and Torrance, C. (2000) 'Written drug dosage errors made by students: the threat to clinical effectiveness'. *Clinical Effectiveness in Nursing*, 4: 20–29

Whittaker, N. (1987) 'Finding the right answer'. *Senior Nurse*, 6(6): 33

Wick, G. (2006) 'PURAT: Is clinical judgement an effective alternative?'. *Wound UK*, 2(2): 14–24, in: Stephen-Haynes, J. (2006) 'Implementing the NICE pressure ulcer guideline'. *Wound Care*, September S16–S18

Woodrow, P. (2004) 'Arterial blood gas analysis'. *Nursing Standard*, 18(21): 45–52

World Health Organization (2005) Body Mass Index **www.euro.who.int/nutrition/ 20030507_1** (accessed 3 January 2008)

Wright, K. (2005) 'An exploration into the most effective way to teach drug calculation skills to nursing students'. *Nurse Education Today*, 25: 430–36

Wright, K. (2006) 'Barriers to accurate drug calculations'. *Nursing Standard*, 22(20): 41–5

Young, T. (2004) 'Guidance on pressure ulcer risk assessment and prevention'. *Nursing Times*, 100(14): 52–3

Index